BRAGG

WATER

THE SHOCKING TRUTH
That Can Save Your Life!

THE WATER YOU ARE DRINKING
MAY LOOK PURE AND SAFE . . .
BUT IS IT?

Blessings of Health

PAUL C. BRAGG, N.D., Ph.D.
LIFE EXTENSION SPECIALIST

and

PATRICIA BRAGG, N.D., Ph.D.
HEALTH & FITNESS EXPERT

Patricia

Health   *Peace*
Happiness   *Youthfulness*
Love   *Joy*
Praise   *Patience*
Vitality   *Fortitude*
Strength   *Charity*
Faith

JOIN
Bragg Health Crusades for a 100% Healthy World for All!

HEALTH SCIENCE
Box 7, Santa Barbara, California 93102 USA

World Wide Web: www.bragg.com

Notice: Our writings are to help guide you to live a healthy lifestyle and prevent health problems. If you suspect you have a medical problem, please seek alternative health professionals to help you make the healthiest informed choices. Diabetics should fast only under a health professional's supervision! If hypoglycemic, add Spirulina or barley green powder to liquids when fasting.

BRAGG

WATER

THE SHOCKING TRUTH
That Can Save Your Life!

PAUL C. BRAGG, N.D., Ph.D.
LIFE EXTENSION SPECIALIST

and

PATRICIA BRAGG, N.D., Ph.D.
HEALTH & FITNESS EXPERT

Health Science, Box 7, Santa Barbara, California, 93102

Telephone (805) 968-1020, FAX (805) 968-1001

To see Bragg Books, Products and health tips on-line,
visit our World Wide Web Site at: www.bragg.com
e-mail address: bragg@bragg.com

Quantity Purchases: Companies, Professional Groups, Churches, Clubs, Fundraisers, etc. Please contact our Special Sales Department.

This book is printed on recycled, acid-free paper.

- REVISED AND EXPANDED -
Copyright © Health Science

Twenty-Eighth printing MCMXCVIII
ISBN: 0-87790-063-9

Published in the United States
HEALTH SCIENCE, Box 7, Santa Barbara, California 93102 USA

PAUL C. BRAGG N.D., Ph.D.

Life Extension Specialist • World Health Crusader
Lecturer and Advisor to Olympic Athletes, Royalty and Stars
Originator of Health Food Stores – Now Worldwide

For almost a Century, Living Proof that his
"Health and Fitness Way of Life" Works Wonders!

Paul C. Bragg is the Father of the Health Movement in America. This dynamic Crusader for worldwide health and fitness is responsible for more *firsts* in the history of the Health Movement than any other individual.

Bragg's amazing pioneering achievements the world now enjoys:

- Bragg originated, named and opened the first Health Food Store in America.

- Bragg Health Crusades pioneered the first Health Lectures across America. Bragg inspired followers to open health stores across America and worldwide.

- Bragg introduced pineapple juice and tomato juice to the American public.

- He was the first to introduce and distribute honey nationwide.

- He introduced Juice Therapy in America by importing the first hand-juicers.

- Bragg pioneered Radio Health Programs from Hollywood three times daily.

- Paul and Patricia pioneered a Health TV show from Hollywood to spread *Health and Happiness* . . . the name of the show! It included exercises, health recipes, visual demonstrations and guest appearances by famous, health-minded people.

- He opened the first health restaurants and the first health spas in America.

- He created the first health foods and products and made them available nationwide: herb teas, health beverages, seven-grain cereals and crackers, health cosmetics, health candies, calcium, vitamins and mineral supplements, wheatgerm, digestive enzymes from papaya, herbs and kelp seasonings, and amino acids from soybeans. Bragg inspired others to follow and now thousands of health items are available worldwide.

Crippled by TB as a teenager, Bragg developed his own eating, breathing and exercising program to rebuild his body into an ageless, tireless, pain-free citadel of glowing, radiant health. He excelled in running, swimming, biking, progressive weight training and mountain climbing. He made an early pledge to God, in return for his renewed health, to spend the rest of his life showing others the road to health. He honored his pledge! Bragg's health pioneering made a difference worldwide.

A living legend and beloved counselor to millions, Bragg was the inspiration and personal health and fitness advisor to top Olympic Stars from 4-time swimming Gold Medalist Murray Rose to 3-time track Gold Medalist Betty Cuthbert of Australia, his relative (pole-vaulting Gold Medalist), Don Bragg and countless others. Jack LaLanne, the original TV Fitness King , says, *"Bragg saved my life at age 15 when I attended the Bragg Crusade in Oakland, California."* From the earliest days, Bragg advised the greatest Hollywood Stars and giants of American Business. J. C. Penney, Del E. Webb and Conrad Hilton are just a few who he inspired to long, successful, healthy, active lives!

Dr. Bragg changed the lives of millions worldwide in all walks of life with the Bragg Health Crusades, Books, Tapes, Radio and TV appearances.

BRAGG HEALTH CRUSADES, Box 7, SANTA BARBARA, CA 93102 USA

PATRICIA BRAGG N.D., Ph.D.

Angel of Health and Healing

Author, Lecturer, Nutritionist, Health Educator & Fitness Advisor to World Leaders, Hollywood Stars, Singers, Dancers & Athletes

Daughter of the world renowned health authority, Paul C. Bragg, Patricia has won international fame on her own in this field. She conducts Health and Fitness Seminars for Women's, Men's, Youth and Church Groups throughout the world . . . and promotes Bragg "How-To, Self-Health" Books in Lectures, on Radio and Television Talk Shows throughout the English-speaking world. Consultants to Presidents and Royalty, to the Stars of Stage, Screen and TV and to Champion Athletes, Patricia and her father are Co-Authors of the Bragg Health Library of Instructive, Inspiring Books that promote a longer, vital, healthier lifestyle.

Patricia herself is the symbol of health, perpetual youth and super energy. She is a living and sparkling example of her and her father's healthy lifestyle precepts and this she loves sharing world-wide.

A fifth-generation Californian on her mother's side, Patricia was reared by The Bragg Natural Health Method from infancy. In school, she not only excelled in athletics, but also won honors for her studies and her counseling. She is an accomplished musician and dancer . . . as well as tennis player and mountain climber . . . and the youngest woman ever to be granted a U.S. Patent. Patricia is a popular gifted Health Teacher and a dynamic, in-demand Talk Show Guest where she spreads the simple, easy-to-follow Bragg Healthy Lifestyle for everyone of all ages.

Man's body is his vehicle through life, his earthly temple . . . and the creator wants us filled with joy & health for a long fruitful life. The Bragg Crusades of Health and Fitness (3 John 2) has carried her around the world over 10 times – spreading physical, spiritual, emotional, mental health and joy. Health is our birthright and Patricia teaches how to prevent the destruction of our health from man-made wrong habits of living.

Patricia's been a Health Consultant to American Presidents and British Royalty, to Betty Cuthbert, Australia's "Golden Girl," who holds 16 world records and four Olympic gold medals in women's track and to New Zealand's Olympic Track and Triathlete Star, Allison Roe. Among those who come to her for advice are some of Hollywood's top Stars from Clint Eastwood to the ever-youthful singing group, The Beach Boys and their families, Singing Stars of the Metropolitan Opera and top Ballet Stars. Patricia's message is of world-wide appeal to people of all ages, nationalities and walks-of-life. Those who follow the Bragg Health Books and attend the Bragg Crusades world-wide are living testimonials . . . like ageless, super athlete, Jack LaLanne, who at age 15 went from sickness to Total Health!

Patricia Bragg inspires you to Renew, Rejuvenate and Revitalize your life with "The Bragg Healthy Lifestyle" Seminars and Lectures worldwide. These life-changing events are where millions have benefitted with a longer, healthier life! Patricia would love to share with your community, organization, church groups, etc. Also, she is the perfect radio and TV talk show guest to spread the message of super healthy living.

For Radio interview requests and info write or call (800) 446-1990
BRAGG HEALTH CRUSADES, BOX 7, SANTA BARBARA, CA 93102, USA

DEADLY HAZARDS OF FLUORIDATED WATER

Forty-one of the 50 largest cities in the U.S. have fluoride, a hazardous waste, in their water. Millions of gallons of this deadly poison are doing untold, irreparable damage by mass medicating everyone who drinks fluoridated water. Let's get this toxic chemical out of America's water supply! If the water in your area is fluoridated, join or start action groups to remove this dangerous chemical now to save yourself, your family and the lives of future generations!

Here are just a few of the serious health problems caused or worsened by fluoridated water:

- Cancer in all its deadly forms.
- Digestive system disorders:
  Ulcers, colitis, constipation, nausea, cirrhosis, hepatitis and inability to utilize vitamins B and C.
- Kidney, bladder and urinary disorders.
- Respiratory and lung disorders:
  Tuberculosis, asthma, rhinitis, sinusitis and bronchitis.
- Circulatory diseases:
  Arteriosclerosis, heart failure, varicose veins, coronary thrombosis, hypo-tension and hypertension.
- Blood conditions:
  Leukemia, hemophilia and anemia.
- Mental and neurological impairments and disorders:
  Neuroses and psychoses, polio and multiple sclerosis.
- Eye diseases:
  Cataracts, vision problems, glaucoma and detached retina.
- Endocrine dysfunctions:
  Diabetes, goiter, and impaired function of the adrenal, thyroid and sex glands.
- Skin, nail and hair conditions:
  Acne, boils, dermatitis, eczema, alopecia and lupus.
- Bone and joint conditions:
  Osteoporosis, bone cancer, arthritis, swollen and aching joints.
- Teeth and gum diseases:
  Mottled and darkened teeth, calcium and bone loss.
- Premature and still births, hearing loss and headaches.

The kind of water you drink can make or break you – your body is 70% water!

THIS BOOK CAN SAVE YOUR LIFE!

More Shocking Facts on Deadly Fluoridated Water:

- Fluoridation is mass drug medication.
- Fluorides are toxic to pets, animals and humans.
- Fluorides are deadly poisons – in the same class as arsenic.
- Fluorides endanger people who drink a lot of water.
- 1 ppm fluoride added to water causes urinary output to increase 3ppm in 24 hrs, overburdening the kidneys.
- Fluorides impair the proper metabolism of fats, carbohydrates, proteins and all food eaten.
- Fluorides are cumulative poisons and some serious side effects may not become evident for 20 years or more.
- Fluorides also affects the genes of 2nd and 3rd generations.
- Fluorides depress the immune system, opening the body to disease and health problems.
- Fluoride passes through the placenta and can harm the baby.
- Fluorides interfere with the metabolism of calcium.
- Fluorides can stunt the growth of all living things.
- The U.S. Government strictly regulates the shipping of products containing sodium fluoride.
- Fluorides are concentrated in processed, canned, bottled and dried foods and can cause grave health problems.
- Not enough is known about how fluoride metabolizes.
- Fluorides in the water can ruin photographic films.
- Fluoridation interferes with all living, growing things.
- Measuring the concentration of fluoride in water is very difficult and often inaccurate.
- The equipment used to fluoridate water is expensive while its repair & replacement is a constant, costly problem.

Important, Vital Water Facts To Know:

- Water is more important than food or vitamin supplements. You can go days without them, but you can't survive long without water!
- 30% of Americans drink water that violates federal health standards!
- More than 90% of water companies don't use available technology to remove chemical contaminants and toxins from drinking water!

Guard Your Health & Life by Drinking Pure, Distilled Water!

This Book Was Written to Alert the World to the Importance of Pure Water to Health

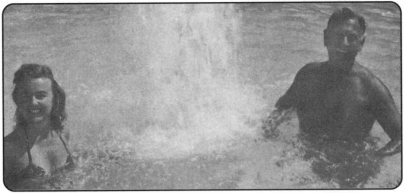

Paul C. Bragg and his daughter, Patricia, bathing in the bubbling fountain of mineral waters in Desert Hot Springs, California. They believe in mineral spas for swimming and bathing therapy, but strongly advise against the use of mineral water for cooking and drinking!

Next to Oxygen, Pure Water is the Most Vital Factor to the Survival of Life!

Humans have survived for as many as 90 days without food, but can live only 72 hours without water before going into a semi-comatose state. Ironically, the kind of water consumed, along with the lack of sufficient water is one of the major substances that brings about arteriosclerosis, illness and premature ageing! Drinking water saturated with inorganic minerals – magnesium carbonate, calcium carbonate and other elements the body cannot use – causes suffering from a variety of unhealthy conditions. Inorganic minerals, toxic chemicals, toxins and contaminants can pollute, clog up and even turn tissues to stone throughout your body, causing pain, illness and even premature death! Distilled water – Mother Nature's flushing agent – helps remove inorganic mineral deposits and toxins from the joints and also helps remove cholesterol and fat from the body. This book unlocks the mysteries of chronic suffering and explains why so many die before their time! Over 80 years of intense research has gone into this book.

3 John 2   Blessings of Super Health and Long Life,

Patricia Bragg   Paul C. Bragg

i

BRAGG HEALTH CRUSADES for the 21st CENTURY
Teaching People World-Wide to Live Healthier, Stronger Lives for a Better World

We love sharing, teaching and giving, and you can share this love by being a partner with Bragg Health Crusades World-Wide Outreach. Bragg Crusades is dedicated to helping others! We feel blessed when your life improves through our teachings from the Bragg Books and Crusades. It makes our years of service so worthwhile!

The Miracle of Fasting book has been the No. 1 book for the past 12 years in Russia. Why? Because we show them how to live a healthy, wholesome life for less money, and it's so easy to understand and follow. Most healthful lifestyle habits are free (good posture, clean thoughts, plain natural foods, exercise and deep breathing that draws energy into the body). We are continuing with all our health teachings, lectures, Crusades, radio, TV and video outreaches to reach you and the world.

My joy and priorities come from God and healthy living. I'm excited about spreading health worldwide, for now it's needed more than ever! My father and I were also TV Health Pioneers, with our program "Health and Happiness" filmed in Hollywood. It's thrilling to be a Health Crusader and you will enjoy it also. See back pages to list names (yourself, family, friends) who you think would like to receive free Health Bulletins!

By reading the Bragg Self-Health Books you can also gain a new confidence that you are helping yourself, family and friends to Healthy Principles of Living! Please call your local health store and bookstore and ask for the Bragg Health Books. Prayerfully, we hope to have all stores stock these books so they will be available to everyone.

I have visions of **Health Retreats** where people can find radiant health, joy and rebirth! They will be **Recharging - Physically, Mentally, Emotionally and Spiritually.** I was reared on Retreats. Holidays and vacations were spent at Camp for precious weeks of growth, and recharge. Everyone needs retreats now, more than ever! You will love them too!

For the new millennium, we are planning Bragg Recharge Retreats and Child & Senior Care Centers which are desperately needed across America. We are just waiting for the right locations and funding. We greatly appreciate all gifts, monetary and land (appraised value), and we can give a receipt for tax deductions. We could develop seldom-used ranches, farms and old estates into Recharge Centers for rejuvenating mind, body and soul. Those attending would become health crusaders for their families and friends. Empty buildings and spacious older homes with yards would make ideal Child & Senior Centers. If you have a location and would like to be part of this great outreach, please call or write to me.

We are not new to retreats: my Dad pioneered the first health spa (Macfadden's Deauville) in Miami Beach and others in Highland Springs, California, and Danville, New York.

I expend all my energy and funds inspiring and helping others to help and heal themselves! Genuine love seeks ways to express itself! I thank you for your caring, sharing support – with your help we can achieve our future goals! I know God will bless you. Your needed help will be a blessing to The Bragg Health Crusades. Our budget is for a mighty worthwhile cause. I know you, your family and friends will enjoy and benefit from our teachings and health retreats.

With A Loving, Grateful Heart, *Patricia Bragg*

BRAGG HEALTH CRUSADES, America's Health Pioneers

A non-profit organization. Gifts are tax deductible.
7340 Hollister Ave., Santa Barbara, CA 93117 USA (805) 968-1020

Over 85 continuous years spreading health and fitness worldwide.

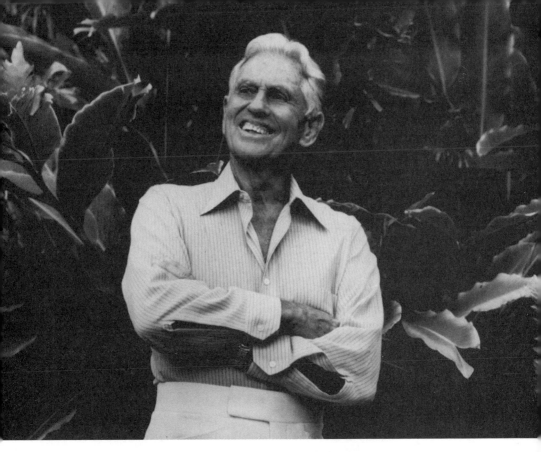

PAUL C. BRAGG, N.D., Ph.D.
World's Leading Authority on Pure Water

Paul C. Bragg's daughter Patricia and their wonderful, healthy members of the Bragg *Longer Life, Health and Happiness Club* exercise daily on the beautiful Fort DeRussy lawn, at world famous Waikiki Beach in Honolulu, Hawaii. Membership is free and open to everyone who wishes to attend any morning – Monday through Saturday, from 9 to 10:30 am – for Bragg Deep Breathing and health and fitness exercises. On Saturday there are often health lectures on how to live a long, healthy life! The group averages 75 to 125 per day, depending on the season. From December to March it can go up to 200. Its dedicated leaders have been carrying on the class for over 27 years. Thousands have visited the club from around the world and carried the Bragg health and fitness message to friends and relatives back home. When you visit Honolulu, Hawaii, Patricia invites you and your friends to join her and the club for wholesome, healthy fellowship. She also recommends you visit the outer Hawaiian Islands (Kauai, Hawaii, Maui, Molokai) for a fulfilling, healthy vacation.

To maintain good health, normal weight and increase the good life of radiant health, joy and happiness, the body must be exercised properly (stretching, walking, jogging, running, biking, swimming, deep breathing, good posture, etc.) and nourished wisely with natural foods. – Paul C. Bragg

iii

Many Waters Contain Deadly Chemicals!

With the scrupulous precision of a responsible scientist, Paul C. Bragg along with his daughter Patricia, describe the serious and devastating dangers in drinking ordinary water loaded with deadly commercial chemicals, toxins and inorganic minerals.

They reveal why the chlorination of our public water supplies may not be the innocent practice that it appears to be. Just remember that chlorine – nascent and the hypochlorite, chlorine dioxide and other chlorine compounds – are strong oxidizing and bleaching agents. When the chlorination of our drinking water is sufficient to produce an offensive taste and smell, enough chlorine may enter the intestinal tract to destroy the friendly bacteria which aid in production and absorption of vitamins, minerals and nutrients.

The Braggs tell you about artificially fluoridated drinking water which 67% of Americans (human guinea pigs) have flowing from their taps . . . an unprecedented experiment which less venturesome nations are watching with growing alarm. **Reread inside front cover warning list.**

They explain how salt (inorganic sodium) causes health problems. Their wise advise is to avoid table salt.

The Braggs believe they have found the reason why we have more hospitals, nurses, mental institutions, medical doctors and other healers, and more medical colleges than ever before in history!

They believe they have found one major reason why so many people are dying of degenerative diseases – such as heart trouble, arthritis, kidney trouble and hardening of the arteries long before their time. In the U.S. rates of Alzheimer's disease, developmental disabilities and deformities are higher than ever before.

From start to finish, this book is enthralling . . . a highly disturbing and immensely serviceable book. It provides life-saving, wise advice. This book is a source of positive and practical enlightenment for everyone who is vitally interested in the methods of regaining and maintaining good health! It shows the way to be healthier, happier and more youthful – plus you will learn how to add energetic years to your life!

Read this book and discover some revealing facts about yourself, your health and your chances of enjoying a longer, more vital life for many years to come!

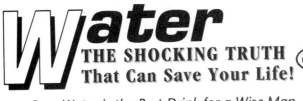

Water
THE SHOCKING TRUTH
That Can Save Your Life!

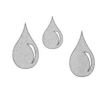

Pure Water is the Best Drink for a Wise Man.
- Henry Thoreau

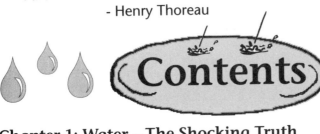

Contents

The best service a book can render you is to impart truth,
but to make you think it out for yourself. – Elbert Hubbard

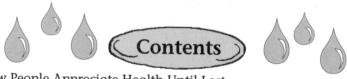

Contents

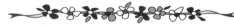

When you sell a man a book you don't just sell him paper, ink and glue, you sell him a whole new life! There's heaven and earth in a real book. The real purpose of books is to trap the mind into its own thinking. – Christopher Morley

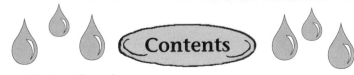

Contents

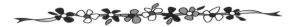

*If a man can convince me that I do not think or act right, gladly will I change,
for I search after truth. But he is harmed who abideth on still in his ignorance.*
– Marcus Aurelius, Roman Emperor

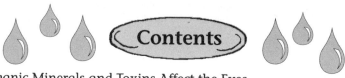

Contents

I have found that distilled water is a sovereign remedy for my rheumatism. I attribute my almost perfect health largely to distilled water. – Dr. Alexander Graham Bell, *Telephone Inventor*

Contents

No horse gets anywhere until he is harnessed. No steam or gas ever drives anything until it is confined. No Niagara is ever turned into light and power until it is tunneled. No life ever grows great until it is focused, dedicated, disciplined. – Harry Emerson Fosdick

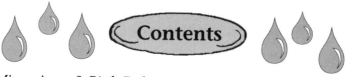

Contents

TEN HEALTH COMMANDMENTS

Thou shall respect and protect thy body as the highest manifestation of life.
Thou shall abstain from all unnatural, devitalized food
and stimulating beverages.
Thou shall nourish thy body with only Natural unprocessed, live foods,
that . . .
Thou shall extend thy years in health for loving, charitable service.
Thou shall regenerate thy body by the right balance of activity and rest.
Thou shall purify thy cells, tissue and blood with healthy foods,
pure fresh air and sunshine.
Thou shall abstain from all food when out of sorts in mind or body.
Thou shall keep all thoughts, words and emotions pure, calm and uplifting.
Thou shall increase thy knowledge of Nature's Laws, follow them,
and enjoy the fruits of thy life's labor.
Thou shall lift up thyself, friends and family by obedience to
God's Healthy, Pure Laws of Living.

Paul C. Bragg   *Patricia Bragg*

Chapter 1

Water – The Shocking Truth That Can Save Your Life!

Pure Water (H_2O) is the Essential Fluid of Life Required for Health!

The most important factors that make for a healthier, happier, longer life are:

- Pure, unpolluted air and practicing deep breathing.
- Drinking pure distilled water that is free from harmful chemicals, toxins and inorganic minerals. Ideal is 8 glasses per day for body maintenance and health.
- Eating natural, organically grown foods is best.

The two most important substances on this earth are air and WATER! Water is perhaps the single most characteristic substance of our planet. It may simultaneously appear in solid, liquid and gaseous forms. It has been adapted as a unit of measure for the specific gravity of all other substances. Water plays important roles in the circulation of the earth's surface elements.

Man must have water or he soon dies! Consider the shipwrecked sailor on a great ocean of salt water – if this man does not get fresh salt-free water, he dies. The man who gets lost in the dry, hot desert soon dies of dehydration if he does not get water. Thirst can drive him insane before he endures an agonizing death.

Certain animals – squirrels, rabbits, etc. that feed on grasses and herbs containing about 85% water never need a drink as long as they can find their natural food.

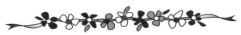

The Law of Cause and Effect: *An unhealthy lifestyle produces illnesses and disease. Most humans are lacking sufficient water intake to maintain optimum body health! Fact: most people are dehydrated most of their lives! It's vital to have 8 glasses of distilled water daily to operate the body functions and achieve The Bragg Healthy Lifestyle for supreme health!* – Paul C. Bragg

The World's Water Supply

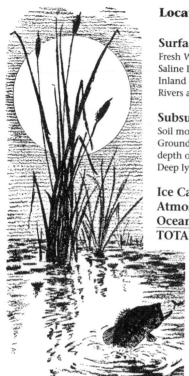

Location	Water Volume (cubic miles)	Percentage of Total Water
Surface Water		
Fresh Water Lakes	30,000	.009
Saline Lakes and Inland Seas	25,000	.008
Rivers and Streams	300	.0001
	55,300	.017
Subsurface Water		
Soil moisture	16,000	.005
Groundwater within depth of half a mile	1,000,000	31
Deep lying groundwater	1,000,000	31
	2,016,000	.625
Ice Caps and Glaciers	7,000,000	2.15
Atmosphere	3,100	.001
Oceans	317,000,000	97.2
TOTAL (approx)	**326,000,000**	**100**

Water is distributed in great or small amounts to every part of the earth. All but about 3% of the water is held in oceans; the remainder is found as deep as 3 miles under the earth's crust or as high as 7 miles above the surface, as vapor. The table above shows the quantity and percentage of water in all its habitats.

Mother's milk contains about 87% water; juicy fruits and succulent vegetables also possess almost the same percentage of fluid. Those who consume ample amounts of fresh fruit daily absorb, in addition to about 8 ounces of solid food, at least 3 pints of living, naturally purified water, distilled by Mother Nature.

Water is one of the most important substances on the face of the earth. Without it, all life – from plants to humans to animals – would cease to exist!

Water Goes On Forever

Water is absolutely indestructible, but unfortunately easily polluted! Scientists believe that there is not a drop more – nor a drop less – than when shallow water first formed the roundness of the earth with its tidal currents. Volcanic eruptions eventually brought solid rock and earth above the water in the form of mountains. Over time, these became the continents.

These tides, conversely, slow the rotation of the earth by a fraction of a second every thousand years. The 24 hour day was probably a 4 hour day millions of years ago. Originally the earth probably consisted of hot gases. As it cooled, hydrogen and oxygen atoms fused to form a steamy mist. Much later, the steamy mist fell in endless torrential rains, the coolness of which eventually solidified the floor of the earth.

The Endless Wonders of God-Given Water

Water shapes the earth, controls the climate and provides man with food and a prodigious amount of energy. The body is 70% water, which is the source of all life, performs and supports the internal body functions of humans and animals and maintains plant life!

It is possible that a tear – which fell from the eye of Jesus when he learned his friend Lazarus had died – has been recycled by the warmth of the sun millions of times and may now repose in the holy water fountain of some obscure church.

3

Water Penetrates Everywhere

The molecular strength of a drop of water is almost beyond comprehension. Penetrating the lacy roots of a big tree, it climbs upward, pulling after it a chain of water drops. The wind will vaporize the water in the topmost leaves of the tree, carrying it back to the sky to help form a rain-bearing cloud. The same drop may be carried as much as 7 miles above the earth, remaining airborne and becoming purified before dropping with billions of other drops as rain . . . perhaps on an orchard of apples. Or the raindrop (distilled water) may be caught by a group of thirsty sailors shipwrecked on a waterless island. It may fall on the parched ground of Arizona and bring to life a seed that needs only a few days of water to grow. An inch of rain that falls over a square mile of topsoil adds over 17 million gallons of water to the earth.

Water is the essential fluid of life . . . the solvent of our ills and the deliverer of a radiant long life.

The Hydrologic Cycle

Rain Clouds

Cloud Formation

PRECIPITATION

while falling

from vegetation

from vegetation

transpiration

EVAPORATION

from streams

from soil

transpiration

from ocean

Surface Runoff

Infiltration

Soil

Percolation

Rock

Deep Percolation

Ground Water

Ocean

One such raindrop, if it lingers on the surface of the earth, may be revaporized and head for the sky in less than a minute. If it penetrates deeply into the ground and enters the water table far below the Sahara Desert, where 150,000 cubic miles of water lies waiting, it may require a century to resurface and become airborne. A solitary drop of water is a strange world indeed.

Hot Mineral Water Under California Desert

Just a few hundred feet below our desert home in California, there is a raging river of hot mineral water. Wells are sunk down to reach this water, which comes out at a temperature as high as 180 degrees. This water has been underground for centuries. The water is cooled to a temperature that human beings can tolerate and provides blessed relief to thousands who have aches and pains throughout their bodies. This warm mineral water is very relaxing and therapeutic. People come from all over the world to bathe in its natural, healing warmth!

We both have painless bodies, yet still take the time to enjoy these hot mineral baths because they are soothing and relaxing to the body and are good preventive medicine. This is the reason we built a home in this spa town – we go to our desert retreat when we want to relax, write and get away from big cities.

Angel View Crippled Children's Hospital in Desert Hot Springs is world-famous for the miracles it's doing with handicapped children. It's an inspiration to see them swimming in the hot mineral water therapeutic pool! Even though many of the children cannot walk when they arrive, they soon learn how to swim in the pool and this starts to build their self-confidence in their little bodies! This hydrotherapy, plus physical therapy, has worked miracles under the pioneering guidance of our good friend, Dr. Frank Edmundson. Our late President and friend, Dwight D. Eisenhower, served on the Board of Directors of this hospital for years.

Niagara Falls is Committing Slow Suicide

Years ago, engineers diverted the Niagara Falls water to study ways of stopping the slag erosion. Man cannot stop the powerful forces of water! Niagara drops 3,500,000 gallons of water over the falls every second. Scientists say that in approximately 20,000 years, this waterfall will retreat to Lake Erie and become a level river.

Our Oceans and Seas

The oceans hold 97.2% of all the water on earth. They create the enormous tides, waves and winds which crash and slam against the rocky beaches and reduce them to sand. Where volcanic eruptions have flowed to the sea, this volcanic material is reduced to sand over time. That is why the Isles of Hawaii and Tahiti have some beaches of black sand. The sea will always win this battle with the earth! Geologists tell us that eventually the mountains will be leveled and swept into the ocean and the cycle of volcanic eruptions will begin again.

Eons ago, continent-spanning glaciers were so numerous that the level of the seas fell 300 feet and land bridges appeared between England and France. An earthen bridge also emerged between Siberia and Alaska. That may account for some of the mystifying similarities among races, even though widely separated by oceans.

Mother Nature is man's teacher. She unfolds her treasures to his search, unseals his eyes, illuminates his mind and purifies his heart. – Alfred B. Street

The famed oceanographer, Columbus Iselin, chided science when he wrote, "The sea is producing about as much as the land, yet man is using only about 1% of his food from his salt water environment." Unfortunately, man is more interested in the unknown darkness of outer space than studying and protecting our vast seas!

Man Cannot Live Without Water

Your existence on earth depends on WATER! Please do not take it for granted! This book gives you an education on the type, amount and value of the perfect water to drink that will work to keep you in good health. Distilled water helps you every day to enjoy a more vital, joyous and prolonged life on our precious earth!

The Five Big Health Builders
• Air • Water • Sunshine • Food • Exercise

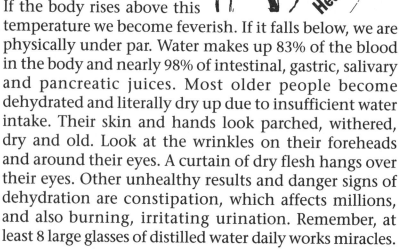

Next to oxygen, water is the most vitally important substance in the body. The adult body is roughly 70% water and excretes water daily through the urine, defecation, perspiration and breathing. The internal temperature of the body is controlled with water.

The average body is 98.6°. If the body rises above this temperature we become feverish. If it falls below, we are physically under par. Water makes up 83% of the blood in the body and nearly 98% of intestinal, gastric, salivary and pancreatic juices. Most older people become dehydrated and literally dry up due to insufficient water intake. Their skin and hands look parched, withered, dry and old. Look at the wrinkles on their foreheads and around their eyes. A curtain of dry flesh hangs over their eyes. Other unhealthy results and danger signs of dehydration are constipation, which affects millions, and also burning, irritating urination. Remember, at least 8 large glasses of distilled water daily works miracles.

The 70% Watery Human

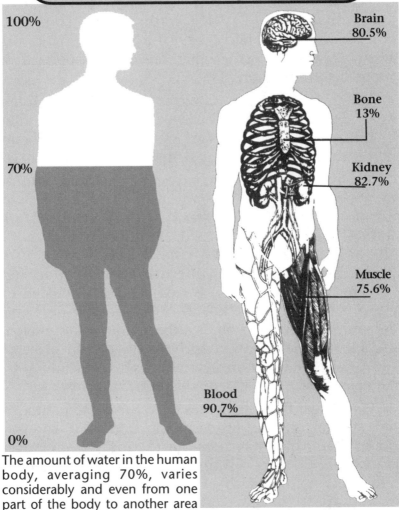

100%

Brain
80.5%

Bone
13%

70%

Kidney
82.7%

Muscle
75.6%

Blood
90.7%

0%

The amount of water in the human body, averaging 70%, varies considerably and even from one part of the body to another area (illustration on right). A lean man may hold 70% of his weight in body water, while a woman – because of her larger proportion of water-poor fatty tissues – may be only 52% water. The lowering of the water content in the blood is what triggers the hypothalamus, the brain's thirst center, to send out its familiar urgent demand for a drink of water.

Water Percentage in Various Body Parts:

Teeth	10%	Lungs	80%
Bones	13%	Brain	80.5%
Cartilage	55%	Bile	86%
Red blood corpuscles	68.7%	Plasma	90%
Liver	71.5%	Blood	90.7%
Muscle tissue	75%	Lymph	94%
Spleen	75.5%	Saliva	95.5%

Water is Important to Superb Health

People who ingest a sufficient amount of the right kinds of liquids (distilled water, fresh fruits and vegetables and their juices) have better body functioning and circulation overall, which are most important to Super Health and Long Life.

You have 15 billion powerful brain cells which are 74.5% water. We strongly believe the right kind of water in sufficient amounts helps improve your mind and brain power and makes you think better and more accurately!

We also think that the excessively nervous and/or mentally upset person is so obsessed with his own worries and "hang-ups" that he just forgets to drink sufficient pure water. Instead, he dopes himself with alcohol, tea, coffee and cola drinks which only complicate his nervous condition by introducing burning, toxic acid into his stomach with no food or water to dilute it. So on top of his nervousness and depression, he suffers from heartburn, sour acid stomach, gas, bloating, enervation and low energy. In place of sufficient pure water, he again dopes up on stimulants, coffee, soft drinks, cigarettes, aspirin, antacids, etc.

Remember that the nerves need the correct amount of water to function properly and smoothly. You can plainly see that it is possible to suffer from water starvation. Here is a simple way that you can help yourself to better health – the Natural Pure Water Way!

The specific reason we wrote this book was to give you the knowledge to select the right kind and amount of water your body so desperately needs! Here is your invitation to enjoy the gift of Super Health, Longevity and Freedom from bodily miseries through following Mother Nature's and God's Eternal Laws combined with the powerful self-health knowledge you are reading.

Shocking Mutations & Death from Polluted Water Must Stop!

Deadly chemical pollution is not only mutating but killing millions of wildlife, fish, etc. worldwide. One USA example: Children in Minnesota discovered and caught frogs displaying horrible mutations, including eyes growing on their knees, four hind legs, etc. Scientists have now determined that unidentified toxic chemicals in the pond and ground water caused these terrible mutations!

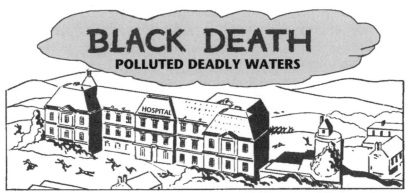

Chapter 2

BLACK DEATH
POLLUTED DEADLY WATERS

The "Black Death" that spread throughout Europe in the 1300s killed one-third of the entire population. This plague was caused by polluted water. Even today in many parts of Europe, the water is unfit to drink. People use bottled water for drinking purposes. Experienced world travelers drink purified bottled water.

"Water! Water! Everywhere – But Not a Safe Drop to Drink!"

Yes, with all the billions of gallons of fresh, sweet water there is on earth, only a fraction of it is fit to drink. A chemical compound known as H_2O, water is one of the most abundant and widely distributed substances on the surface of the earth. It occurs naturally in solid, liquid and gaseous states, generally known as ice, snow, water and steam vapor. Water, composed of hydrogen and oxygen, is contained in varying amounts in all natural foods. It's an indispensable solvent needed in all physiological functions in every form of life.

The body requires water that is 100% pure hydrogen and oxygen, free of toxins and inorganic minerals. This water comes from three sources: **first**, from fresh, organically-grown vegetables and fruits and their juices, which Mother Nature purifies; **second**, from water distilled and purified by steam; **third**, from rain water that comes down through unpolluted, clean air.

Most Americans' bodies thirst for pure distilled water! Their bodies become sick, prematurely aged, crippled and stiff due to inorganic minerals and chemicalized water and lack of sufficient pure water!

Sad fact – much of the world's water today is polluted. It is difficult to find sources of water from rivers, ponds, lakes, streams and even wells and springs which are not polluted or which do not contain traces of toxic industrial chemicals to some degree. Therefore, a great deal of toxic chlorine is added to make this water fit to drink.

But is it really "fit to drink"? Water processing plants use chemical chlorine to destroy the bacteria in polluted water. Alum and many other inorganic chemicals are also used to cleanse polluted water of dirt and filth. See page 124 for some facts about deadly chlorinated water.

In addition to these inorganic chemicals, a dangerous and misunderstood inorganic substance has been added to drinking water – sodium fluoride. It's the worst chemical ever added knowingly to our drinking water; a terrible crime against public health! Please reread inside front cover for startling facts about fluoridation.

Inorganic Versus Organic Materials

Now, let us give you a short lesson in chemistry. There are two kinds of chemicals, inorganic and organic.

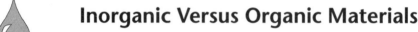

The inorganic chemicals like chlorine, alum and sodium fluoride cannot be utilized in a healthy way by the living tissues of the body and can only cause harm!

Our body chemistry is composed of 19 organic minerals, which must come from a living source or one that was once alive. When we eat an apple or any other fruit or vegetable, that substance is composed of living organic minerals. It has a certain length of life after being gathered from the earth, vine or tree. The same goes for animal foods, fish, milk, cheese and eggs.

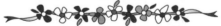

To preserve health is a moral and religious duty, for health is the basis for all social virtues. We can no longer be useful when not well.
– Dr. Samuel Johnson, Father of Dictionaries

Health in a human being is the perfection of bodily organization, intellectual energy and moral power.
– T.L. Nichols, M.D.

Organic minerals are vitally important in keeping us alive and healthy! If we were cast away on a barren, uninhabited island where nothing was growing, we would slowly starve to death. Even though the soil beneath our feet contains 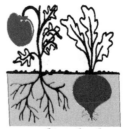 16 inorganic minerals, our bodies cannot absorb them efficiently enough to sustain life. Only a living plant has the power to extract inorganic minerals from the earth and to transform them into useful organic substances to nourish our bodies.

When my father was on an expedition to China many years ago, one part of the country was suffering from drought and famine. With his own eyes he saw poor, starving people heating and eating earth because of the lack of food! They died horrible deaths from starvation, because they could not get the needed nourishment from the inorganic minerals in the dirt.

For years we've heard people say that certain waters were "rich in all the minerals." What kind of minerals are they talking about? Inorganic or organic?

Humans do not have the same chemistry as plants. Only living plants can convert an inorganic mineral into an organic mineral. As you read here, you will learn what harm inorganic minerals can do to your body and brain.

Because of dietary deficiencies, some children and young animals try eating dirt. They can become deathly ill, not from the germs in the dirt, but from the inorganic minerals which can cause sickness and even death!

Old age is a highly toxic condition caused by nutritional deficiencies and an unhealthy lifestyle.

DRINK, DRINK, DRINK. *You can easily sweat away more than a quart of water during an hour of strenuous exercise. Sweat rates of nearly a gallon an hour have been reported in some athletes. For optimal hydration during strenuous endurance exercise, drink at least 16 to 20 ounces of fluid 2 hours before exercising and another 8 ounces 15 to 30 minutes before. While exercising, sip 4 to 6 ounces every 15 to 20 minutes. Afterwards, drink enough to replace the fluid you've sweated off; drink one pint for each pound lost.*

During my father's boyhood on a Virginia farm, his family raised dairy cattle. Salesmen would come to the farm to sell various kinds of feed. Dad remembers when his father purchased cattle food labeled "The Mighty Mineral Cattle Food." It was supposed to have lots of calcium, magnesium and other important minerals to help build strong cows that would produce extra milk. However, all of the minerals in this "mighty" cattle food were derived from powdered limestone and other inorganic sources: calcium carbonate, magnesium carbonate, etc. When this inorganic mineral formula was mixed with organic food, the cattle absolutely refused to eat the feed. Their innate dietary instincts prevented them from eating powdered limestone. All of the neighboring farmers had the same experience. We learned later that this worthless, inorganic mineral cattle food was taken off the market.

Dangerous Inorganic Minerals And Toxins in Our Drinking Water

As previously noted, chlorine, alum and other inorganic minerals such as calcium carbonate, magnesium carbonate and potassium carbonate are used to "purify" our drinking water. Constantly keep in mind that **the human body needs hydrogen and oxygen as a natural solvent in its internal chemistry.** Therefore our bodies need a constant supply of clean water. Where to get it? Even untreated, so-called "pure" water from springs, wells, etc. nearly always contains some traces of inorganic minerals and often other toxic matter.

This is the irony of Mother Nature: that this fluid – without which man can barely exist more than 72 hours before lapsing into a semi-comatose state – contains in most of its forms the exact inorganic chemicals which bring about the ultimate premature ageing of man and animals. And, as stated earlier, the major aluminum companies want to pollute all our water with sodium fluoride, a deadly waste product produced through aluminum processing.

Kids exposed to high levels of fluoride have lower IQs. – Fluoride Magazine

Fluorine is a Deadly Poison

Millions upon millions of innocent people have been brainwashed by the aluminum companies to erroneously believe that adding sodium fluoride to our drinking water will reduce tooth decay in our children. Over 135 million Americans drink a daily dose of sodium fluoride in their water without thinking of it!

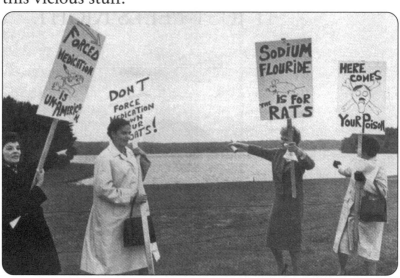

Fluorine, the gangster of the chemical underworld, made the atomic bomb possible. The only scientific way to free the necessary quantities of fissionable Uranium 235, buried in the inert mass of its parent U-238, is to force uranium hexafluoride gas through many acres of porous barriers. The next part of the process gradually concentrates the elements, creating a deadly hazard from radiation. "Hex" is what they named this vicious stuff.

These 11 Associations Stopped Endorsing Water Fluoridation in 1996

- *American Heart Assoc.* • *American Academy of Allergy & Immunology*
- *American Cancer Society* • *Chronic Fatigue Syndrome Action Network*
- *American Diabetes Assoc.* • *National Institute of Law Municipal Officers*
- *American Chiropractic Assoc.* • *American Civil Liberties Union*
- *Nat'l Kidney Foundation* • *American Psychiatric Assoc.* • *Soc. of Toxicology*

Millions of Americans drink water spiked with a sodium fluoride solution. A chemical cousin of sodium, fluorine is not as toxic as "Hex" . . . but toxic enough, in high concentrations, to be used as a standard roach and rat killer and a deadly pesticide.

Yet this terrible, deadly sodium fluoride, injected virtually by government edict into drinking water in the proportion of 1.2 parts per million (PPM), has been declared by the United States Public Health Service to be "absolutely safe for all human consumption". Every qualified chemist knows that such "absolute safety" is not only unattainable, but a total illusion!

The Grim Story Behind Fluoridation

It was in the year 1939 that a famous institute in the eastern part of the United States commissioned their biochemist to find a use for the sodium fluoride wastes produced by aluminum foundries. Some 45 other industries also had fluoride disposal problems. Many were tormented by expensive damage suits arising from the noxious effects of the poison on livestock and crops. Oil refineries, metal smelters, tile, brick, steel, fertilizer and ceramic plants and many installations of the Atomic Energy Commission were involved. The cost to eliminate this chemical was fantastically high. Was there no way this by-product could be put to a profitable use?

Now this biochemist was a clever and cunning man. He came up with a big money-making idea: why not dissolve the stuff in drinking water? He had absolutely no medical background and had not conducted any clinical research into the effects of sodium fluoride on our body's chemistry. His idea went over big with companies who were burdened by what to do with sodium fluoride wastes.

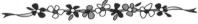

Russian studies in the 1970s demonstrated that workers suffering from exposure to fluoride in the workplace exhibited signs of impaired mental functioning. – Health Action Network

From the British Journal Nature, *1986: Researcher Mark Diesendorf assessed 24 studies from 8 countries and found cavity rates had declined equally in fluoridated and nonfluoridated areas, showing fluoridation isn't necessary!*

The USA leads the world in heart diseases, strokes, cancers and diabetes!

The next step was not difficult . . . turn the idea over to the advertising companies and let them brainwash the public into believing that the greatest health measure in modern times had been discovered. Give a "tall tale" to the gullible American public and if it sounds scientific, they will bite – hook, line and sinker! So they used the tall tale that sodium fluoride in drinking water would prevent tooth decay in children, as they found a Texas town that had naturally occurring fluoride and it seemed fewer dental cavities. The public was eager to hear more. At last, a way to prevent tooth decay! Sadly, most became convinced at first – despite that every smart thinking person knows that tooth decay comes from poor nutrition and especially the high consumption of refined sugar drinks, candy and products.

Big business and large professional organizations have a way of sticking together. Remember, they have the power of the media behind them because of the economic control exerted by the publishers' chief source of income – advertising! With the aid of television, radio, newspapers and magazines, the major business, professional and social organizations promoted the 'great merits' of sodium fluoride – although totally false and dangerous – to the American people.

17

Any person who publicly questioned this poisoning of drinking water with sodium fluoride was called stupid, ignorant, uninformed and backward! Most doctors and dentists surrendered to these powerful forces for fear of being discredited by their professional associations and communities. However, you can always find some honest and sincere professionals who fight for truth – no matter how others might ridicule them! Extreme pressures were put upon city and state governments to fluoridate the drinking water. Big business and large professional organizations, which can act like the Mafia, do not take "No" for an answer! They know how to pressure state, city and water officials to think and take action their way, often not for good!

Health risks associated with our current fluoride intake (exceeds 6 mg/day) can be described in a nutshell: An intake of 5 mg/day will cause average individuals to develop crippling deformities of the spine and major joints within a lifetime.

Shocking Historical Fluoride Facts

- Adolf Hitler sought a means to make people docile and suggestible. He discovered that odorless sodium fluoride slowly poisons and makes dormant the small tissue in the brain's left rear occipital lobe that normally helps a person resist domination. Fluoride allows muscles to move one way, but not relax. In large doses fluoride causes paralysis and death.

- Sodium fluoride is classified with arsenic and cyanide as a dangerous poison and is used in rat poison. Hydrogen fluoride is an industrial pollutant. It is illegal to sell or give away a fluoride pill of 1 mg. Fluoride slowly destroys the body's self-repair and rejuvenation capabilities causing premature ageing, bone damage and deformities.

- Fluoride increases the risk of hip fractures up to 41%. Fluoridation can cause tooth enamel mottling, poor health, mongolism in infants and increases the growth of cancer cells.

We all must demand safe, pure water!

The Fluoridation Fiasco*

- In recent years, fluoridation of our water supply has been shown not only ineffective in preventing tooth decay, but it poisons the body! How and why should public health policy and the American media live with and perpetuate this toxic sham?

- At first, industry could dispose of fluoride legally only in small amounts by selling it to insecticide and rat poison manufacturers. Then a commercial outlet was devised in the 1930s when a connection was made between water supplies bearing traces of fluoride and lower rates of tooth decay. Even after this connection was proven erroneous, it became a political, not a scientific issue. Many opponents originally started out as proponents, but changed their minds after closer looks at mounting evidence. They started viewing it as a capitalist-style con job of epic proportions poured down American throats.

* Excerpts from an article by Gary Null called The Fluoridation Fiasco.

More Fluoridation Fiasco Facts:

- The Sierra Club found in a study that people in unfluoridated developing nations have fewer dental caries than those living in industrialized nations. They concluded "fluoride is not essential to dental health."

- In British Columbia, only 11% of the population drinks fluoridated water, as opposed to 40-70% in other Canadian regions. Yet British Columbia has the lowest rate of tooth decay in Canada, with the lowest rates of dental caries occurring in areas of the province where the water is not fluoridated.

- In 1986-87, 39,000 school children between ages 5 and 17, living in 84 areas around the country were studied. ⅓ of the places were fluoridated, ⅓ were partially fluoridated and ⅓ were not. Results showed no statistically significant differences in dental decay rates between fluoridated and unfluoridated cities.

- A World Health Organization survey reports a decline of dental decay in Western Europe, which is 98% unfluoridated. Europe's declining dental decay rates are equal to and sometimes lower than U.S. rates.

- A 1992 University of Arizona study yielded surprising results when they found that "the more fluoride a child drinks, the more cavities appear in the teeth."

- All Native American Indian reservations are fluoridated by law. Children living on them have more incidences of dental decay and other oral health problems, caused by high sugar, refined foods, etc., than do children living in other U.S. communities.

- Most of Western Europe has rejected fluoridation on the grounds that it is unsafe. Sweden's Nobel Medical Institute recommended against fluoridation and the process was banned. The Netherlands outlawed the practice in 1976. France decided against it after consulting with its Pasteur Institute. West Germany, now Germany, rejected the practice because 1 ppm was dangerously "close to the dose at which long-term damage to the human body is to be expected."

The noblest of the elements is water. – Pindar

More Fluoridation Fiasco Facts:

- J. William Hirzy, Ph.D., Senior Vice-President, National Federation of Federal Employees stated in a letter, July 2,1997 to Jeff Green, of Citizens for Safe Drinking Water, "I am pleased to report that our union, which represents and is comprised of the scientists, lawyers, engineers and other professionals at the headquarters in Washington, D.C. of the US Environmental Protection Agency, has voted to co-sponsor the California citizen's petition to prohibit fluoridation. The evidence over the last 11 years indicates a causal link between fluoride and cancer, genetic damage, neurological impairment, bone pathology and lower IQ in children. We conclude that the health and welfare of the public is NOT served by the addition of fluoride to the public water supply!"

- Some fruit juices contain shocking amounts of fluoride, with some brands of grape juice containing much higher levels – up to a highly toxic 6.8 ppm! The use of fluoride-containing insecticides in grape crops is a factor in these high levels. Cooking can greatly increase a food's fluoride content. Also, keep in mind that toxic fluoride is an ingredient in pharmaceuticals, aerosols, insecticides and pesticides. Common fluoride levels in toothpaste are 1000 ppm. When fluoride is ingested, approximately 93% of it is absorbed into the bloodstream and what is not excreted is deposited in the bones and teeth.

- Fluoride use is absolutely unsafe and should be stopped immediately! The government feels that its central concern is to protect industry, therefore the solution to pollution is dilution! You poison everyone a little bit rather than poison a few people a lot. This way, people don't know what's going on. Any public health official who criticizes the practice of fluoridation is at risk of losing his job. Even National Toxicology Program researchers downgraded cancers caused by fluoridation after being coerced by superiors to change their findings.

Some students drink deeply at the fountain of knowledge. Others only gargle. – Paul C. Bragg

- Fluoride has been proven to cause osteosarcoma, a rare bone cancer; squamous cell carcinoma in the mouth; fluorosis of the teeth; osteosclerosis of the long bones; liver cancer; chromosome aberrations; genetic damage; and skeletal fluorosis and deformities. B. Spittle, author of *Psychopharmacology of fluoride: a review* states "There appears to be evidence that chronic exposure to fluoride may be linked with cerebral impairment affecting particularly concentration and memory in some individuals."

More Fluoride Warnings!*

Studies show that fluoride in all its uses, including public drinking water, causes cancer:

- The overwhelming evidence shows that fluoridation is causing an increase in bone cancer and deaths among males under 20.

- The growing increase in bone cancer attributable to fluoridation may all be due to also an increase in osteosarcoma caused by fluoride.

- The overall preponderance of evidence shows that fluoridation is causing an increase in oral (mouth) cancer among human populations. Don't use fluoride toothpastes or give your dentist consent to do fluoride gel treatments or use fluoride polishing paste.

- Fluoride has been linked to many health problems:
  • bone and oral cancers in animals and humans
  • an ability to inhibit the DNA repair enzyme system
  • it accelerates tumor growth • it inhibits the immune system • it causes genetic damage in a number of different cell lines and induces melanotic tumors, fibrosarcomas, etc. • other tumors and cancers strongly indicate that fluoride has a generalized effect of increasing them overall.

- According to our estimates, over 10,000 people in the United States die of cancer each year due to fluoridation of public drinking water.

* Excerpted from Fluoride, the Aging Factor by Dr. John Yiamouyiannis.

The best method for purifying your water is a system that distills your water and then carbon filters it. – Dr. Robert Willix, Jr.

More Shocking Fluoride Updates!

● **Hip Fracture Rate Highest in U.S.**
The fluoridation of our water is weakening our bones, slowly but surely.
– U.S. National Research Council and Townsend Letter for Doctors

● **Fluoride and Osteoporosis**
Seniors living in areas with elevated fluoride levels in drinking water suffer up to 41% more hip fractures. In a study of 3,578 senior citizens, those who lived in areas with fluoridated water had a much greater risk of hip fractures.
– Journal of the American Medical Association

● **Fluoride and Bone Cancer**
One study concluded that males under the age of 20 who live in areas with fluoridated water were six times more likely to suffer from bone cancer than males who don't. – New Jersey Department of Health

● **The Deadly Costs of Fluoridation**
When a claimed 20% decrease in tooth decay is compared to a 600% increase in bone cancer or a 41% increase in hip fractures, when the cost of a tooth filling is compared to the cost of a hip fracture or cancer treatment, it is obvious that the human and economic costs of fluoridation are staggering.
– Health Action Network

● **Fluoridated Water Increases Bone Cancer Risk**
In a study conducted by the New Jersey Department of Health, young men who drank fluoridated water had a higher incidence of bone cancer. – The Record

22

● **Osteoporosis, Calcium and Fluoride**
The National Institutes of Health (NIH) gathered a panel of "experts" to discuss the causes of the rising epidemic of bone fractures in the elderly. Although the evidence clearly shows that calcium supplements don't help, and just as clearly shows that fluoride is terrible for the bones, the NIH simply recommended an increase in the recommended daily allowance of calcium.
– The Fluoride Report

● **The Overwhelming Evidence that Fluoride Weakens Bones**
Dr. John Lee showed that "...7 out of 10 recent studies show a clear correlation between bone fractures and water fluoridation. One of these studies involved 560,000 women over 65. The size of this study completely obliterates the few reports of small populations that showed no correlation."
– The Fluoride Report, September, 1994

● **Fluoride Actually Reduces Bone Strength, Instead of Increasing It!**
In a five year study conducted to test fluoride as a treatment for osteoporosis, bone density was actually decreased 45%, therefore causing osteoporosis, rather than preventing it! The doses used were very close to the amount Americans take in over a fifty year span. – Bone, Vol. 15, 1994

● **How The EPA is Spending Your Tax Dollars**
When Dr. Bill Marcus won back his job with the EPA after being fired for blowing the whistle on the cover-up of fluoride's hazards, the EPA refused to pay interest on his two years of lost wages. While the lawyers haggle, the whole sum is being withheld, and guess who's paying for the EPA's lawyers?
– The Fluoride Report

More Shocking Fluoride Updates . . .

- **Fluoridation Accidents Swept Under the Rug**
Toxic spills of fluoride in drinking water have happened in several communities, but these were never publicized. Nausea, vomiting, diarrhea and even deaths occurred. – Townsend Letter for Doctors

- **Why Do Researchers Continue to Support Deadly Fluoridation?**
Once accepted, scientific theories become very hard to debunk. Research done on the topic after a theory has been accepted becomes "a strenuous and devoted attempt to force nature into the conceptual boxes supplied by professional education."
– Thomas Kuhn, The Structure of Scientific Revolutions

- **Fluoride: Shocking Facts**
Fluoride has never received FDA approval and wouldn't pass if it were subjected to the FDA's standards of safety and effectiveness. It's more toxic than lead by the EPA's standards and accumulates in the body. The maximum allowable lead in drinking water: 0.015 mg/liter; the maximum allowable for fluoride: 4.000 mg/liter. – Health Action Network

- **Fluoridation: A Health Violation of Medical Ethics**
Fluoride is a pharmacologically active substance unrelated to water purification. There is no possibility of obtaining individual informed consent for medication with this experimental drug when it is placed in a public water system. For these reasons, fluoridation violates the Nuremburg Code of medical ethics and human rights. – Health Action Network

- **Fluoride: Industrial Waste**
The fluoride in your water is actually toxic waste left over after the manufacture of aluminum and chemical fertilizers.
– Dr. John Yiamouyiannis, *Fluoride, the Aging Factor*

- **Environmental Protection Agency Infighting**
EPA toxicologists have long been asking that the standards for water fluoridation be revised, while EPA administrators continue to reject their warnings and have even disciplined employees who have spoken out. – The Pittsburgh Press

- **Fluoridation is Big Business**
Despite the fact that it doesn't actually prevent tooth decay in children or adults, government officials still devote our tax dollars to fluoridation. Several other countries tried it and stopped when their research showed that the risks far outweighed the benefits. In this country, the big companies that make huge profits from selling this toxic waste material are so powerful that the facts are swept under the rug. – Let's Live! May 1996. This magazine, originally called California Health News, was started by Paul C. Bragg, who changed the name because, he said, "Everybody wants to – Let's Live!"

- **Mohawk Indians' Fluoride Tragedy**
In the period from 1960 to 1975, a Mohawk Indian tribe in the Northeast U.S. was all but obliterated by fluoride contamination. Cows, fish and children all suffered from tooth and bone deformities caused by wastes from two major metals manufacturers. (Now all Indian reservations have fluoridated water!)
– "Fluoride: Commie Plot or Capitalist Ploy?" by Joel Griffiths

23)

More Shocking Fluoride Updates . . .

- **Fluoride is Highly Toxic**

The fact is that fluoride is more toxic than lead and just slightly less toxic than the killer arsenic. – Gary Null, *The Fluoridation Fiasco*

- **Use Non-Fluoride Toothpaste**

Fluoride in toothpaste is absorbed through the lining of the mouth, and in only one or two brushings, a milligram of fluoride enters your body.
– Health Action Network

- **Fluoridation Increases Lead Contamination**

Fluoride leaches lead from plumbing and water mains. In Tacoma, Washington, where lead content of water had risen above EPA limits, fluoridation was halted because of equipment failure. Officials were surprised at the resulting 50% drop in lead contamination.
– Letter from C.R. Myrick, Water Quality Coordinator, Tacoma, WA

- **Fluoride Affects Immune Function**

Because of its disabling effects on enzyme activity, fluoride reduces resistance against infection. – Complementary Medical Research

- **Fluoride Adversely Affects Central Nervous System**

Scientific studies link fluoride to learning disabilities and coordination problems.
– Townsend Letter for Doctors

- **Fluoride and Decreasing Birth Rates**

Fluoride is found to decrease fertility in studies of animals and humans.
– Journal of Toxicology and Environmental Health

- **Highly Publicized Fluoride Studies Show Medical Mistake**

The high doses of sodium fluoride used in clinical studies of this drug are known to lead to a condition called osteofluorosis. This means abnormal bone growth and calcification of tendons and ligaments. Although this may help prevent spinal fracture and compression, it also increases risk of hip fracture and causes arthritis-like pain.
– Open letter from John Lee, M.D., to C.Y.C. Pak, M.D., regarding Dr. Pak's study on sodium fluoride in the *Annals of Internal Medicine*

- **Juice Drinks Contain Dangerous Levels of Fluoride**

42% of prepared juices contain toxic levels of fluoride. Grape juice is especially bad because of the fluoride-containing insecticides used on grapes.
– Journal of Clinical Pediatric Dentistry

- **Danger is Not Only in The Water But in Processed Foods**

There are no regulations on fluoride content of processed foods. Many of these packaged foods are loaded with deadly fluoride. – Health Action Network

- **Tooth Decay Decline Unrelated to Fluoride**

Tooth decay has declined worldwide, with no difference between countries with or without water fluoridation. – Health Action Network

God will not change the condition of men, until they change what is in themselves. – Koran

More Shocking Fluoride Updates . . .

● **The Sad, Unnecessary Epidemic of Dental Fluorosis**
This disease, marked by tooth enamel malformation, mottled-discoloration and brittleness, affects up to 30% of children living in areas with fluoridated water. Only 10% of children in non-fluoridated locations have dental fluorosis.
– Public Health Service figures

● **H. Dean Changes His Mind and Retracts Fluoridation Endorsement!**
H. Trendly Dean, the original promoter of water fluoridation, admitted under oath in 1955 that it doesn't work as a remedy for tooth decay.
– Fluoride, Vol. 14, No. 3, July 1981

● **Study Reveals That Fluoride Causes Tooth Decay**
Children in India who drank fluoridated water suffered from significantly more tooth decay than children who did not. Especially at risk were children with very little calcium in their diets.
– The Journal of the New Zealand Pure Water Association

● **Children Poisoned by Toothpaste**
When fluoride toothpaste was first sold in the 1950s, warnings that it should not be used in children under six were eliminated from the package – because they damaged sales! When two children in Tacoma, Washington, began to throw up every night before bed, doctors told the parents that their toothpaste was to blame. At last fluoride danger warnings are mandatory on all new fluoride toothpaste labels! – The Fluoride Report

There are hundreds of case histories of people who have overcome health problems when they began drinking distilled water.
– Dr. Clifford Dennison Ed.D., *Why I Drink Distilled Water*

Chronic Fatigue Syndrome sufferers are instructed to drink distilled water.
– Dr. Edward M. Wagner, *How to Stay Out of the Doctor's Office*

We have time enough if we will use it right. – Johann W. Goethe

Keep Toxic Fluoride Out of Your Water!

Most water Americans drink has fluoride in it, including tap, bottled and canned drinks and foods! Now, ADA (American Dental Assoc.) is insisting that the FDA mandate the addition of fluoride to all bottled waters! Defend your right to drink pure, nonfluoridated tap and bottled waters! Challenge and stop local and state water fluoridation policies! Call, write, fax or e-mail your state officials and conrgess people and send them a copy of this book.

CHECK FOLLOWING WEB SITES FOR FLUORIDE UPDATES:

- ● www.bragg.com   ● www.citizens.org
- ● www.sonic.net/~kryptox/fluoride.htm
- ● www.cadvision.com/fluoride/index.htm
- ● emporium.turnpike.net/P/PDHA/fluoride/fluor.htm
- ● www.garynull.com/documents/fluoridation.htm
- ● users.aol.com/forgood/swis

Danger – Don't Drink Water Contaminated with Sodium Fluoride

Fluoride is one of the most potent poisons known to man. Selling this poison swells the bank accounts of the big companies who, in turn, pay big dividends to their stockholders. This money is made by selling a waste by-product! All these industries had to do, using the media and powerful lobbies, was brainwash the public into accepting their false statements that fluoride added to their water would prevent tooth decay.

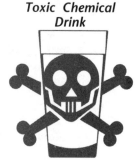
Toxic Chemical Drink

Now the drinking water in most cities is being fluoridated due to the powerful organizations who are sponsoring this mass poisoning. In our opinion, many early deaths today are caused by premature damage to our arteries due to sodium fluoride. Fluoride can also damage the heart, lungs, liver, brain and other vital organs; not only the arteries!

Read and reread this book carefully! More than 85 combined years of research has gone into acquiring and compiling this vital information for your health.

Who wants to return to the old days when food had a taste and water didn't and you couldn't even see the air you breathed? The realization of the deterioration of the environment and of problems of population, food, power and water, has been growing on us through a frightening total of isolated reports. Penguins accumulate DDT in Antarctica, the California redwood forests are going fast, there are power blackouts in major cities, lead enters the atmosphere from gasoline – contributing to smog, there is mercury in the rivers, radioactive waste and nerve gas are dumped into the oceans. Every newspaper and news magazine worldwide brings another bad situation to the reader's attention and there are crises everywhere. No matter what the real situation is, the constant bombardment creates a feeling of hysteria and despair. – Water: The Web of Life by Robert M. Garrels & Cynthia A. Hunt

In contemplating the nature of water I feel that it is the mother, the life of all material manifestation. It is the most flexible and yet the most solid, the most destructive but, next to air, the most necessary. No matter how much it is mixed with other substances, when we distill it, it is cleansed and purified into clean distilled water so that we can drink it to our benefit.
– Jeanne Keller, Healing with Water

We Live in a Sick, Sick World

We are independent researchers and health crusaders for the truth. We're loners. No one controls what we say. No organization dictates to us! We have no financial master to serve; therefore we can give you the plain, honest truth. We love inspiring and guiding you with our simple, easy-to-follow Bragg Healthy Lifestyle, so you can enjoy a long, vibrantly youthful life! We've spent our lives researching and studying human health. We've been trying to understand why people become sick, prematurely old, senile and die long before their time!

It's our conclusion that many make themselves sick and shorten their lives by consuming unhealthy toxic water and unhealthy foods! Plus, many use tobacco and consume powerful stimulants such as alcohol, coffee, tea and sugared colas. They eat also high concentrations of refined white sugar and its products, refined white flour products such as white bread, pasta, white rice, salt and salted foods. They overeat and eat refined, dead

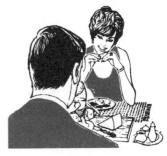

Foods can make or break your health. You can dig your grave with your knife, fork and spoon!

devitalized foods and too much meat and saturated fats! These are the killers that fill the arteries with waxy, clogging cholesterol.

These bad, unhealthy habits – plus lack of exercise, sunlight and fresh air – add up to physical unfitness. 97% of people today are physically unfit and 65% are overweight. Most people eat such an unhealthy diet that they suffer from sickness and fatigue. They drag around all day and at night are forced

We are a nation of pill takers. Every 24 hours between 50 and 75 tons of pain killers and other so-called remedies are consumed.

to take a sleeping pill to sleep. When they awaken they take a "pep pill" to stay awake and keep them going!

Physical fatigue and weariness make them more inactive than ever. They just don't have the "Go Power" to lead active physical lives. As a consequence, their exterior as well as interior muscles suffer from increasing flabbiness. The greatest "disease" today is the physical deterioration of the human body at all ages.

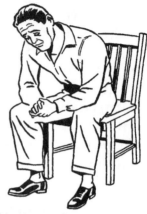

Let's take a good, hard look at our young people. Never in the entire history of the world have so many drugs been used by people under thirty! Why do young people turn to drugs to keep them going? Just take a look at the "junk" and "trash" they eat – that tells the entire sad story! They do not derive

This picture shows a victim of chronic fatigue. He has no energy, vitality, strength or ambition. He suffers from extreme weariness physically and mentally, which is a state of physical deterioration.

28

enough nutrients, vitamins and minerals from their daily diet! In their ignorance, they try to gain energy by using harmful stimulants such as coffee, sugared drinks, tobacco, alcohol and drugs. These deficient, "dope addicts" are in danger of having children who are born sickly and some with breathing and birth defects!

Few People Appreciate Health Until Lost

For many people, health is something they value only when they have lost it or are in danger of losing it. We repeat, "We live in a sick, sick, world – and it's getting sicker every day!" Take heed, repent and change now!

"Health" is an old Anglo-Saxon word meaning "soundness." The ancient Greek concept of "a sound mind in a sound body" *(mens sana in corpore sana)* gives the true picture of health. We have to place the adjective "good" with this word "health" only when we contrast it with the phrase "ill health" or "lack of soundness."

The natural healing force within you is the greatest force in getting well.
– Hippocrates, Father of Medicine, 400 B.C.

A healthy, energetic body and an alert, keen, healthy mind make it possible for human beings to cope with and bear the frustrations, worries, cares, tensions and stresses of life and yet enjoy life and the joys of this world . . . even as confused, feverish and mixed-up as it is today! Where there is vigorous health, there is not even an awareness of the complex mechanisms and chemistry that go on inside of us to make this possible. Within our bodies, the most magnificent chemical and mechanical procedures known and unknown to man are carried on.

We take our health for granted, as we do the moon and the sun – usually even neglecting to be thankful. We get up in the morning after a sound night's sleep, ready to take on the day's work and expect to end the day comfortably tired. It's best to earn your sleep with work and exercise – then you will sleep better for sure!

Marvelous Mechanisms of the Body

If we had transparent skin and could look inside ourselves, we would see the lungs taking air into their delicately fashioned chambers. If we smoked, we would see tobacco's vicious nicotine and tars coating these pink, beautiful, healthy organs to a sticky, deadly black. **If you smoke – stop now! The strong survive longer!**

We would see the heart receiving blood through numerous intricate channels from the billions of our body's cells and pumping it out, refreshed and purified, by another route back to these same tissues. We would get an exact picture of our arteries, veins and capillaries. We could see how much corrosion is taking place because of our consumption of the heavy inorganic minerals and toxic chemicals that are put into our drinking water. If we could examine our arteries closely, we would see that calcium carbonate and its associates are lining these pipes and making them brittle – beginning to literally turn our bodies into stone. Oh, if everyone could see what inorganic minerals do to the arteries – they would be sure to follow the wise advice given in this book! Remember, we are as young as our arteries!

Men do not die; they kill themselves. – Seneca, Roman Philosopher

If we could look inside ourselves, we would also see the digestive tract performing miraculous changes to the foods and drinks we consume. We would see it transform salads, raw nuts, seeds, raw and cooked organic vegetables, fruits and other healthy foods into vital substances our bodies' cells need and can use. People who live on dead, devitalized diets would see how the body's chemistry struggles to handle hot dog

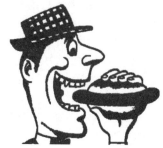

Nitrates and nitrites are harmful food additives.

sandwiches, processed deli meats, commercial ice cream, doughnuts and all the other "food trash" that insults, sickens and clogs their digestive tracts and bodies!

If we could get a full view of the largest organ in the body, the liver, we would see how it struggles to handle alcohol, coffee, tea, cola, soft drinks and other unhealthy liquids. We would see the disastrous effects of the dangerous inorganic chemicals that are added to our drinking water

by man. Also, Mother Nature can often do more harm than man by contaminating water with inorganic minerals such as calcium, magnesium and potassium carbonates and many other substances. Looking closely, we would see that the liver is hardening into stone.

Thousands upon thousands of people die from a disease known as cirrhosis of the liver – fibrosis, which is a hardening caused by excessive formation of connective tissue followed by contraction of the liver. Both hard water's inorganic minerals and alcohol consumption hardens the liver. The world is recklessly consuming alcohol products which is leading to grave health problems – please drinkers, beware and stop!

The health journals all agree that the best and most wholesome part of the doughnut is the hole. The larger the hole, they say, the better the doughnut.

To fare well implies the partaking of such food as does not disagree with body or mind. Hence only those fare well who live temperately. – Socrates

Autonomic Nervous System
– The Body's Communication Network –

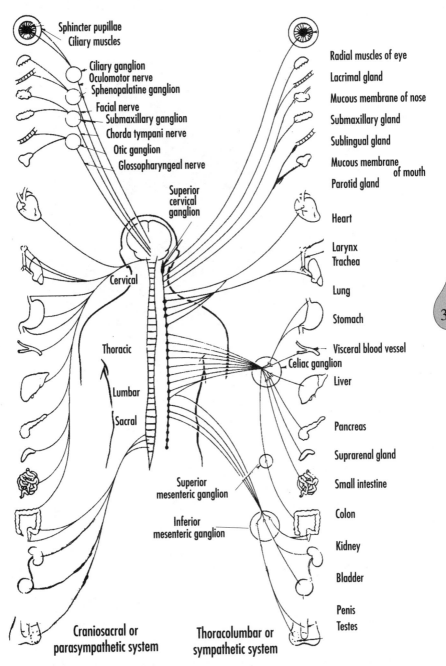

Sphincter pupillae
Ciliary muscles

Ciliary ganglion
Oculomotor nerve
Sphenopalatine ganglion
Facial nerve
Submaxillary ganglion
Chorda tympani nerve
Otic ganglion
Glossopharyngeal nerve

Superior
cervical
ganglion

Cervical

Thoracic

Lumbar

Sacral

Superior
mesenteric ganglion

Inferior
mesenteric ganglion

Craniosacral or
parasympathetic system

Thoracolumbar or
sympathetic system

Radial muscles of eye
Lacrimal gland
Mucous membrane of nose
Submaxillary gland
Sublingual gland
Mucous membrane of mouth
Parotid gland

Heart

Larynx
Trachea

Lung

Stomach

Visceral blood vessel
Celiac ganglion
Liver

Pancreas

Suprarenal gland

Small intestine

Colon

Kidney

Bladder

Penis
Testes

31

Autonomic Nervous System, showing its 2 divisions:
the craniosacral or parasympathetic, and
the thoracolumbar or sympathetic systems.

THE DIGESTIVE SYSTEM

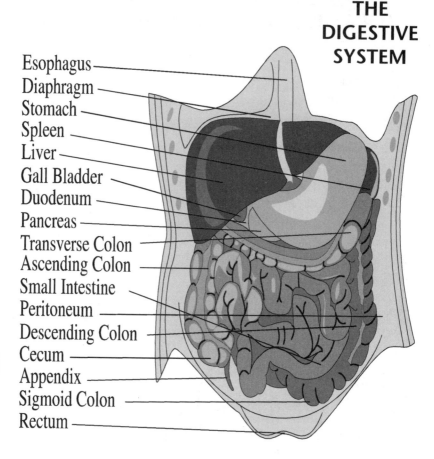

Esophagus
Diaphragm
Stomach
Spleen
Liver
Gall Bladder
Duodenum
Pancreas
Transverse Colon
Ascending Colon
Small Intestine
Peritoneum
Descending Colon
Cecum
Appendix
Sigmoid Colon
Rectum

Your Body's Many Cries for Water;
You Are Not Sick, You Are Thirsty.
These powerful quotes are from the book by F. Batmanghelidj, M.D.

- *Pure water is a natural medication for a variety of health conditions.*

- *Chronic cellular dehydration can painfully and prematurely kill. Its initial outward manifestations have until now been labeled as diseases of unknown origin.*

- *For the process of digestion of food, water is the most essential ingredient. If the body has the necessary water in it before we eat food, the battle against cholesterol formation in the blood vessels might be won.*

- *Cholesterol production in the cell membrane is a part of the cell survival system. It is a necessary substance. Its excess denotes dehydration.*

- *Pure water is the cheapest form of medicine to a dehydrated body.*

Hardening of the Arteries

On several occasions during my father's boyhood in Virginia, his parents took him to the famous Luray Limestone Caverns. There he saw how, drop by drop, water loaded with limestone slowly formed the stalactites and stalagmites over eons of time. These were huge formations created by deposits of the inorganic minerals that are ever-present in most drinking water.

Calcium carbonate, or lime, is a very important ingredient in making cement or concrete. This catalytic agent is responsible for the hardening of concrete. When taken into the body chemistry and subjected to the process of natural metabolism through the years, this mineral becomes the principal troublemaker responsible for what is called "hardening of the arteries." Doctors call this degenerative arterial condition "arteriosclerosis," and most people believe it to be a natural condition that comes with the passing of the years. This is "herd mentality" thinking – or rather, non-thinking! Very few people question this age-old superstition. Many people accept the fallacy that they must face arteriosclerosis and senility in their golden years. Read on – be informed.

Normal Artery Compared to Clogged Artery

Normal Artery   **Clogged Artery**

These photomicrographs show (A) a normal artery seen in cross section and (B) a diseased artery in which the channel is partially occluded by atherosclerosis.

Exercise reduces the risk of heart disease through both direct effects on the cardiovascular system as well as through reduction of intra-abdominal fat. Therefore, the goal of exercise and maintaining normal weight should be to lower the potential for cardiovascular disease.

The very finest doctors will assert that there is no known cure when hardening of the arteries takes place. New techniques have been developed to implant plastic arteries in place of the larger arteries and veins of the heart and the neck. There is expensive heart vascular surgery and also expensive surgical procedures for cleaning out the inorganic deposits of some of the larger arteries of the body. But when you consider the extent of the entire pipe system of the human body, cleaning out a small amount could not accomplish a great deal. Miles of arteries, veins and capillaries would have to be cleansed of their inorganic crust to be effective. Read on – there is a solution to stop this hardening: practicing The Bragg Healthy Lifestyle!

Brains Turned to Stone

The greatest damage done by inorganic minerals – plus waxy cholesterol and salt (sodium chloride) – is to the small arteries and other blood vessels of the brain. It also causes deterioration of the kidneys, liver, heart and other vital organs of the body. Essentially, premature ageing and senility are the brain turning into stone! Visit the large convalescent and rest homes and see with your own eyes the number of people who can no longer reason or think for themselves. Many of them cannot even recognize their own children and relatives!

Millions of people have lost all power of thinking! They often have no control over their eliminative organs and have to wear diapers. Many of them have to be hand fed. All the higher functions of the brain are gone. Their eyes stare into empty space.

This is the way many end up! Millions are saved from this tragedy because they die before their body chemistry has time to turn their brains to stone. Hardening of the arteries and calcification of the blood vessels starts the day you are born, because from birth we begin taking inorganic minerals and chemicals into our bodies.

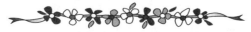

The nervous system falters and suffers when we do not take care of our body.

Miracle Functions of the Human Brain

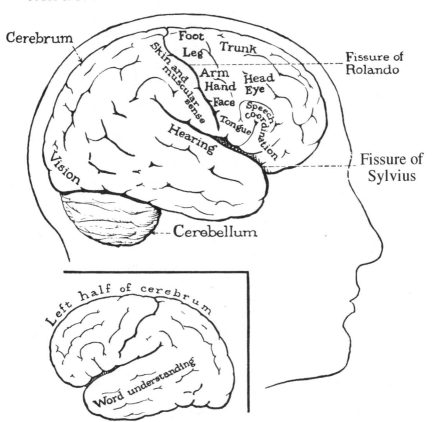

No power on earth can restore the life of a brain hardened by
inorganic minerals that has virtually turned to stone.
Don't let this happen to you! This condition is preventable!
Drink organic vegetable and fruit juices and safe, pure distilled water only.

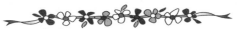

There is a great deal of truth in the saying
that man becomes what he eats. – Gandhi

There is only one water that is clean and that is steam distilled water.
No other substance on our planet does so much to keep us healthy and
get us well as this water does. – Dr. James F. Balch, MD, *Dietary Wellness*

Our prayers should be for a sound mind in a healthy body. – Juvenal

Paul Bragg's work on water and fasting is one of the great contributions to
the Healing Wisdom and the Natural Health Movement in the world today.
– Gabriel Cousens, M.D., author, *Conscious Eating and Spiritual Nutrition*

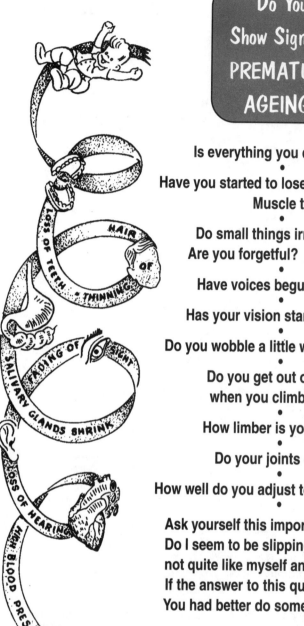

Do You Show Signs of PREMATURE AGEING?

Is everything you do a big effort?

Have you started to lose your skin tone?
Muscle tone?

Do small things irritate you?
Are you forgetful?   Confused?

Have voices begun to fade?

Has your vision started to dim?

Do you wobble a little when you walk?

Do you get out of breath
when you climb stairs?

How limber is your back?

Do your joints creak?

How well do you adjust to cold and heat?

Ask yourself this important question:
Do I seem to be slipping and
not quite like myself anymore?
If the answer to this question is "Yes,"
You had better do something about it!

START TODAY
Living The
Bragg Healthy
Lifestyle!

He who understands nature walks with God. – Edgar Cayce

Chapter 3

Bragg Speaks About His Childhood

Paul C. Bragg's Early Experiences With Hard Water

I was born on a farm in Virginia, along the Potomac River. We got all our drinking water from a well overflowing with crystalline, fresh water. It was very hard water because

it contained a great deal of calcium carbonate and other inorganic minerals from limestone in suspension or solution.

This hard water made laundering and cleaning difficult. The soap used for these purposes simply would not make suds. Water softeners are good to use only for doing laundry and please never use for cooking, food preparations, drinking, etc.

Limestone Water

When we boiled this water, inorganic mineral encrustations formed in large slabs inside the kettles. In time, it created holes in the bottoms of the kettles. Kettle after kettle had to be thrown away, with the same deteriorations happening to each kettle.

But the greatest damage done to humans who drank this hard, inorganic mineral water was to their cardiovascular systems and their overall health.

My grandfather was a man in his mid-sixties. He was a big, strong six-footer – about 200 pounds of solid muscle. My grandfather was a loving Christian family man, an expert horseman and a hard working farmer.

I can remember when he had his first major stroke. There was a large family of Braggs, and we were seated together around the dinner table. Suddenly, there was a crash of dishes when my grandfather slumped over the

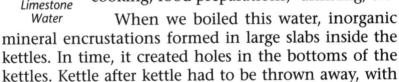

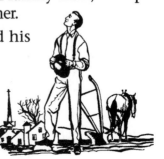

37

Teach me Thy way O Lord; and lead me in a plain path. – Psalms 97:11

table. When the country doctor arrived, he stated sadly that grandfather had lost all control of his left side due to brain damage.

From then on, he needed constant attention. With a completely paralyzed left side, he could not walk without the aid of someone to steady him. He had absolutely no control of his eliminative system. There was great difficulty getting food into his body because he had lost the ability to chew. Only very soft, bland food could be fed to him.

This fine man we knew and loved was, as far as real living was concerned, dead. You have no idea what a great burden he was on my parents and family. The poor, helpless man struggled on in this manner for 3 years. Then the second and final stroke came and he died. The doctors who performed the autopsy stated that his arteries were like stone. My grandfather was born and reared on that farm and drank that hard water every day of his life.

I Discovered the Miseries Caused by Hard Water

I was just a little boy when my father explained to me the outcome of my grandfather's autopsy. I asked my father in despair, "How could his arteries turn into stone?" He couldn't give a satisfactory answer to my question. That very day, I resolved to find out why my grandfather's arteries had hardened.

I read medical books loaned to me by my Uncle William, who was our family doctor. I besieged my uncle with hundreds of questions as to why human arteries could become like stone. It was to be many years before my questions were answered. In the meantime, I witnessed what the hard water was doing to my family, our relatives and friends.

Drinking the right water in the right quantity at the right time is just as important as eating well. Pure distilled water is the right drink! – Paul C. Bragg

Good health and good sense are two of life's greatest blessings. – P. Syrus

Millions Suffer With Joint Pain

Many fine people from all walks of life worked on our farm. We all got along together as one big family. One of the women who worked in our home was named Bessie Louise. She was just like a member of the family, and we all loved her dearly. Poor Bessie developed arthritis in her hands, wrists, elbows, hips, knees and ankles. How that poor woman suffered day after day from tormenting pain! Sometimes the pain would be so great that she would burst into tears.

Again I asked my doctor, Uncle William, what caused the arthritis. I wanted to know if there was a cure for this tormenting condition. He answered me honestly. "Paul," Uncle William said, "we do not know the cause of crippling, painful arthritis, and we have no cure for it. All I can do is give Bessie strong painkillers to relieve her great suffering."

SEVEN TYPES OF JOINTS

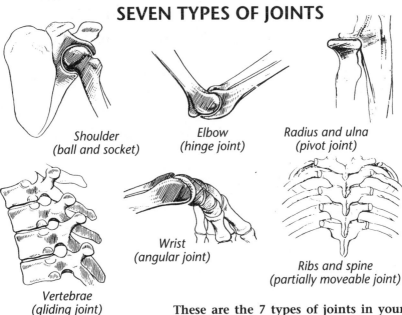

Shoulder
(ball and socket)

Elbow
(hinge joint)

Radius and ulna
(pivot joint)

Vertebrae
(gliding joint)

Wrist
(angular joint)

Ribs and spine
(partially moveable joint)

Cranium
(immovable joint)

These are the 7 types of joints in your body, moveable and immovable. Between each of the moveable joints there is a clear amber fluid called synovial fluid which acts as a lubricant to keep the joints moving freely and easily. When inorganic minerals from drinking water and toxic acid crystals replace this synovial fluid you experience stiffness, pain and misery.

In time, poor Bessie was confined to her bed in pain. In just a few years she was dead. She never reached 65. Her last years were filled with intense pain, misery and suffering.

My poor young brain suffered. "What causes this horrible, crippling disease?" I would ask myself in the late hours before going to sleep.

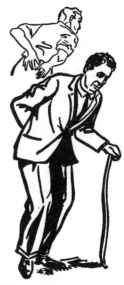

Here we were living on a big, fine farm, with an abundant supply of foods of all kinds. We had a good, comfortable home. It was a beautiful farm on a majestic river. But there was suffering among the adults. These pains were grouped under one

Millions suffer with pain.

word, and that was "misery." Each day I would hear my mother ask different people, "How is your misery today?" The sufferers would answer my mother dolefully.

Frustrated, I would go to our kind and patient doctor, Uncle William, and put the question squarely to him. "Uncle," I would ask, "Why do so many people suffer from the misery?"

His answer was, "I wish I knew." Then again I would say to myself, "Someday, I will find out why people suffer from *the misery!"*

T.B. in My Teens

When I was just a lad I saved a man from drowning. As it turns out this man was very rich and to reward me for saving his life he gave me a scholarship to a large military school. My parents were very eager for me to attend, so at the tender age of 12, I was enrolled in a large military school in the south.

At the military school, I not only drank hard water, but I was fed a poor institutional diet. We were served loads of starches such as refined flour hot cakes, biscuits and white rice. For our meals, we could select several overcooked meats, hot dogs, sausages, fried potatoes, and end up with heavy desserts loaded with white sugar

Locations in the Body where Osteoporosis, Arthritis, Pain and Misery Hit the Hardest

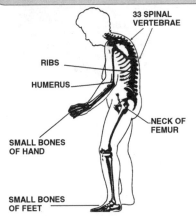

33 SPINAL VERTEBRAE

RIBS

HUMERUS

SMALL BONES OF HAND

NECK OF FEMUR

SMALL BONES OF FEET

OSTEOPOROSIS
Affects 20 Million Kills 300,000 Americans Annually

Boron
Miracle Trace Mineral For Healthy Bones

41

BORON – A trace mineral for healthier bones that also helps the body absorb more vital calcium, minerals and necessary hormones! Good sources are most vegetables, fresh and sun dried fruits, raw nuts, soybeans and nutritional yeast.

The U.S. Department of Agriculture's Human Nutrition Lab in Grand Forks, North Dakota, says boron is usually found in soil and in foods, but many Americans eat a diet low in boron. They conducted a 17 week study which showed that a daily 3 mg. boron supplement enabled participants to reduce the loss (demineralization) of calcium, phosphorus and magnesium from their bodies. This loss is usually caused by eating processed fast foods and lots of meat, salt, sugar and fat and the lack of fresh vegetables, fruits and whole grains in your diet.

After only 8 weeks on the boron supplement, participants' calcium loss was cut 40%. It also helped double the levels of certain important hormones which are vital to maintain calcium and healthy bones. Millions of women on estrogen replacement therapy for osteoporosis may want to use boron as a healthier choice. Also check wild yam Progest cream.*

Scientific studies have shown that women benefit from a healthy lifestyle that includes some gentle sunshine and ample exercise to maintain healthier bones, combined with a low fat, high fiber and carbohydrate diet. This helps protect against heart disease, high blood pressure, cancer and many other ailments. I'm happy to see science now agrees with my Dad who first stated these simple health truths over 85 years ago!

For more osteoporosis and hormone facts read John Lee, M.D.'s book What Your Doctor Won't Tell You About Menopause

including doughnuts, sweet buns, chocolate cakes, pies, puddings, cookies and ice cream.

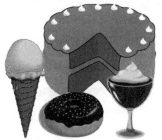

In exactly 4 years, at only 16, I was a sad victim of tuberculosis. Again and again I asked my uncle who was a doctor why this had happened to me. He could not answer my question.

I spent time in several T.B. sanitariums – to no avail – and then fate intervened. I was skin and bones and so sick and weak. When four staff doctors examined me, I asked them point-blank, "Are you going to save me from this disease?" I received an honest answer. "No," they said, "We don't believe you're going to make it."

When they left the room, my human angel – Maria, the Swiss exchange nurse – seemed angry. "These American doctors know nothing about T.B.," she declared. "I am glad I am returning to a sanitarium and a doctor who has cures!" I cried out, "Will you take me to that doctor? I want to live so I may help all sick people! I want to be a Health Crusader!"

42

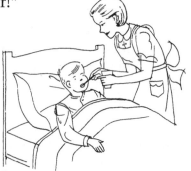

So, the Swiss nurse took me to her wonderful sanitarium in Switzerland where the great physician, Dr. August Rollier, gave me a new life by using all natural healing methods. He administered no drugs of any kind – just distilled (rain) water, good nutrition, sunshine, fresh air, deep breathing, massage and exercise. In 2 years, I was healthy and strong as a young stallion. Now I was ready to achieve my life's ambition of helping others to help themselves to superb health!

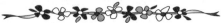

Nature, time and patience are the three greatest physicians. – Irish Proverb

Up to 90% of deaths annually are self-inflicted by unhealthy lifestyle!

Dear friend, I wish above all things that thou may prosper and be in health even as the soul prospers. – 3 John 2

The Secret of Rain and Snow Water: It's Distilled By Mother Nature

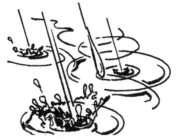

Many of the practices of Dr. Rollier's sanitarium are now standard T.B. treatments. In many ways, this doctor was years ahead of others and his wise health care saved my life!

He was very insistent upon one point: "No hard water should ever be given to a patient." Although water is abundant in Switzerland, Dr. Rollier gave us only water from rain and melted snow (distilled by Mother Nature). He was also a great believer in the use of fresh vegetable and fruit juices.

Dr. Rollier always told us the reasons for his treatments. He explained, "Practically all of the water in Switzerland is *heavy* or *hard* water, loaded with inorganic minerals. This hard water burdens and brings only harm to our bodies, because the body chemistry can assimilate only organic living foods and liquids."

43

I admired, loved and followed Dr. Rollier because he gave logical answers to my questions. What a brilliant man! He brought healing to patients from all over the world who had been doomed to die, including myself. When I left the sanitarium, he cautioned me that I must drink only rain and snow waters, vegetable and fruit juices (all distilled by Mother Nature) and distilled water.

The Answer to Healthful Living

Pondering Dr. Rollier's advice, I thought, "Could it be possible that my grandfather's death from a stroke and Bessie Louise's death from crippling arthritis had a common basis? Was it due to drinking hard water and eating dead, devitalized foods?" These questions nagged at me. I had to find the answers. I felt a great burden; a burden that could be lifted only when I found the truth. Then the answers to such disease and death would no longer be a mystery!

The secret of longevity is eating and drinking intelligently. – Gayelord Hauser

It was then that I pledged to God to be a biochemist, nutritionist and doctor who healed using only natural methods. After I left the sanitarium, I spent 8 years in school and doing research for knowledge which would equip me to help sufferers help themselves to health!

I've been blessed by helping millions to better health and am more enthusiastic than ever about the miracle powers of Mother Nature's healing. That's why my dedicated daughter Patricia and I have written this life-changing book, which is long overdue, for now we have the answers that will save millions from suffering!

My First Two Cases

As noted earlier, after 2 years at Dr. Rollier's sanitarium in Switzerland, I was reborn with a new healthy life! Completely cured of T.B., I was in excellent condition. The Alpine sunshine, the pure rain and snow distilled water to drink, the clean air of the Alps and the natural diet had given me a new body. Every cell in my body vibrated with vigorous health! Now I was ready to study biochemistry and other related health subjects to prepare for my life's work being a health crusader.

Deciding to live and study in London, I found a small apartment not far from the famous Regent's Park. In my opinion, this is one of the most beautiful parks in the world. Here I could take my early morning runs, hikes and play tennis. In my apartment, I could prepare and enjoy my live food meals and fresh juices.

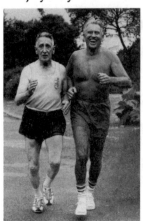

McLean and Bragg

The owner of the building lived on the first floor. He and his wife were typical, prematurely old people. They ate the regular English diet. It contained plenty of refined white flour (bread, biscuits and

Paul C. Bragg and Duncan McLean, England's oldest champion sprinter (83 years young) on a training run in London's famous Regent's Park.

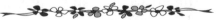

Whatsoever was the father of a disease; an ill diet was the mother. – Herbert

other refined products), large amounts of sugar jams and jellies along with gallons of tea full of sugar and milk. Their vegetables and meats were all overcooked. To top it all, they drank London tap water, which was heavily chlorinated, chemicalized and loaded with calcium carbonate and harmful toxins that cause body stiffness.

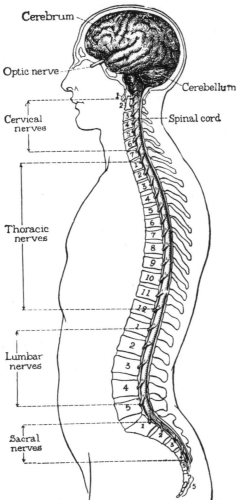

45

General View of the Central Nervous System and Spine

It is in the cushions between the bones of the spine that inorganic minerals from water may deposit themselves and cause painful stiffness, backaches, slipped discs and many other spinal-back problems. Important Nerve Force to the vital organs may then be greatly reduced, causing painful miseries throughout the body.

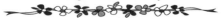

Vegetarians have denser, better formed bones and stronger immune systems.
– Linda Rector Page, N.D., Ph.D., *Healthy Healing*

When I came to inspect the fifth floor apartment – a "walk-up" with no "lift" or elevator – the owner, Mr. Wilson, gave me the key and told me his joints were so stiff that he could not walk up the five flights. So I went up alone and found the apartment to be exactly what I wanted. Among other things to my liking, it was unheated. However, there were small, built-in grates; if I wanted heat, I would have to order coal and have it delivered in bags.

I settled down comfortably in my fifth floor London apartment and started my schooling in biochemistry. My landlords, the Wilsons, were very friendly and from time to time I would drop by their apartment for a visit. Both of these nice English people had numerous physical troubles. Mr. Wilson suffered greatly from low back pain, as well as pains in all his moveable joints and some form of bladder disease. Mrs. Wilson was not much better off. She was 50 pounds overweight and huffed and puffed with every move. She also suffered from kidney disease. During my visits, a good part of our conversation centered around their many ailments.

By this time, the cruel London winter had set in. Outside, it was damp and cold. But each day before dawn, I would put on my heavy sweat clothes and take a long run in Regent's Park, returning to the apartment glowing with good circulation and health. I never had as much as a sniffle all winter, but the Wilsons were plagued with one cold after another. They had large amounts of toxic mucus pouring out and felt terrible most of the winter.

One Saturday, when I stopped by their apartment after my morning run, I could see that Mr. Wilson was desperately ill. He was running a high fever and his nose was so completely stuffed up that he had to breathe through his mouth. I went into his bedroom, which was overheated and had very little oxygen. The poor man looked up at me and said, "For God's sake, you're studying health, help me! I feel so sick – like I'm dying!"

"Mr. Wilson," I told him confidently, "if you will follow the natural system of healing that I will outline for you, you can get well!"

From Sickness to Superb Health

I knew I could help him, but I wondered before making my offer if he was strong enough of mind and wanted to achieve *health* passionately enough?

"I will follow your instructions to the letter," he stated in desperation, like a drowning man grasping a helping hand.

"Good! Today you will start on a 10 day cleansing fast." I picked up the bottles on the bedside table. "Soon all this medication will go down the drain." I brought him some of my distilled water, purchased apple cider vinegar, lemons and honey for him and started him on his first fast day. It was not easy for this man to fast. Mr. Wilson was so full of toxic poisons, so full of sticky mucus in his head, throat and lungs that he had a great deal of discomfort and trouble getting rid of it. But he was an Englishman with plenty of fortitude. He passed a lot of toxic wastes from his body. At the end of the 10 day fast, he felt better than he had for many years!

Then, I put him on a natural live food diet consisting of fresh fruit and vegetable juices and distilled water. Within 3 weeks after his fast, he climbed the 5 flights of stairs to my apartment – something he had not done in 7 years! His wife became enthusiastic about my natural way of living and began to follow the program which became The Bragg Healthy Lifestyle. She started to shed the fat from her body that she couldn't lose before.

After 6 months you could not tell the Wilsons were the same people. They were healthier, stronger and happier! Mr. Wilson ran up to my apartment twice a day. Mrs. Wilson looked trim and slim and had to have all her clothes taken in. Their married daughter lived in Canada and came for visit. She could not believe what she saw. The Wilsons' health troubles were gone. They were now enjoying life fully and it made me happy!

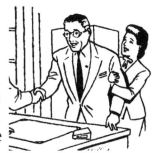

The Wilsons thanked me and said they felt "reborn." By following The Bragg Healthy Lifestyle, they found new, vigorous health.

These were the first two cases who followed my new Bragg Healthy Lifestyle. The results gave me confidence which grew as I studied the teachings of the world's great healers. It was Hippocrates, the father of medicine, in 400 B.C. who gave these wise words to the world to use:

> *Let food be your medicine and medicine be your food.*

Mother Nature's Way

We give thanks for the millions of people who read our books and have come to us for advice through the years and have literally been reborn healthy again by living The Bragg Healthy Lifestyle which is Mother Nature's Way! We feel blessed to know we've inspired people to make positive, healthy changes in their lives.

This is Mother Nature's own natural lifestyle. There is a big difference between feeling well enough to carry on one's daily activities with no sensation of anything wrong, and that more exhilarating state of health which fills one with enthusiasm for life and its challenges. An adequate amount of that important commodity – vibrant health – supplies sufficient energy for life to go on serenely, but it takes more to give one a sense of exuberance. People who live by Mother Nature's Eternal Laws will enjoy an exalted feeling of well being that is not euphoric (abnormally happy and buoyant), but is the result of a natural *joie de vivre* or joy of living.

The Wilsons discovered this joy of living when they changed from their unhealthy lifestyle and went on The Bragg Healthy Lifestyle. They learned through their own experience that the body is a naturally self-repairing and self-healing instrument. Mr. Wilson found out that the stiffness in all his moveable joints was not due to the number of years he had lived, but due to the wrong kinds of food, water and lack of exercise! He learned that time is not toxic, but it's lifestyle and habits that count.

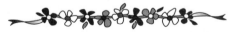

When pure rules of business and conduct are observed, there is true religion. Walk in the path of duty, do good to your brethren and work no evil towards them.

Mother Nature and its beauty is the signature of God. – Patricia Bragg

Mr. Wilson's stiffness was brought on by a combination of toxic acid crystals from an unbalanced, acid diet and drinking water saturated with inorganic minerals and toxic chemicals. Fasting helped to dissolve these encrustations which had been deposited in his joints. A natural diet and distilled water continued the cleansing and healing process and helped prevent a recurrence of his former ailments.

The same thing happened with Mrs. Wilson's weight and kidney problems. She felt remarkably improved. By switching from their old unhealthy ways to The Bragg Healthy Lifestyle – Mother Nature's way – they were able to enjoy their full potential and experience the true joy of healthy living and superb energy!

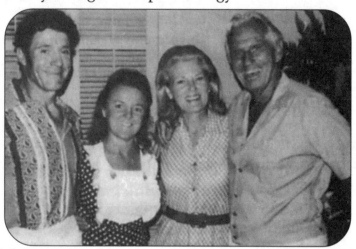

49

Jack LaLanne, Patricia Bragg, Elaine LaLanne & Paul C. Bragg

Jack says, "Bragg saved my life at age 15, when I attended the Bragg Health and Fitness Crusade in Oakland, California." From that day, Jack has continued to live a healthy lifestyle, inspiring millions to health and fitness!

Ponce de Leon

Searched for the "Fountain of Youth."

If he had only known It's within us . . . Created by the food we eat! Food can make or Break your health!

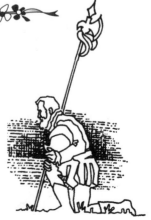

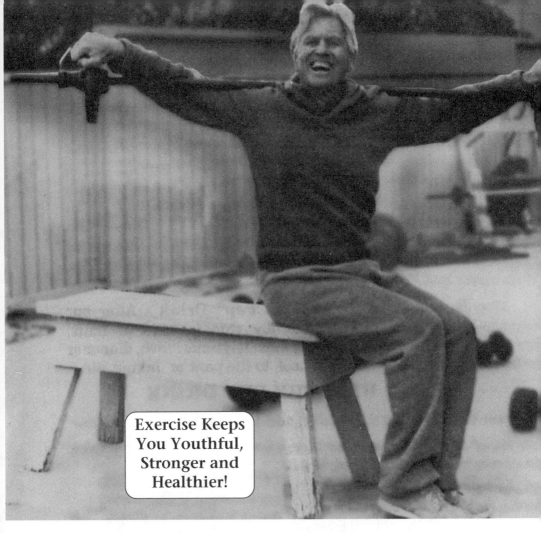

> Exercise Keeps
> You Youthful,
> Stronger and
> Healthier!

Paul C. Bragg and Patricia Lift Weights 3 Times Weekly

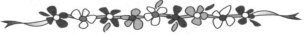

Give us Lord, a bit of sun,
A bit of work and a bit of fun.
Give us, in all struggle and sputter,
Our daily whole grain bread and food.
Give us health, our keep to make
And a bit to spare for others' sake.
Give us too, a bit of song
And a tale and a book, to help us along.
Give us Lord, a chance to be
Our goodly best for ourselves and others
Until men learn to live as brothers.

An Old English Prayer

Chapter 4

Water and Its Effects
On the Human Body

The Stones Within Us

The more we learned about biochemistry (life chemistry), the more we realized why so many people were prematurely old and suffering from pain throughout their bodies. During our visits to London's largest hospitals, we learned more about stones forming within the human body.

Why do stones form in our bodies? What does this mean with regard to human health?

The most common places to find such stones are in the gallbladder, the kidneys, the passageways between kidneys and bladder (known as the ureters) and within the bladder itself. Another organ where stones are sometimes revealed by an X-ray is the pancreas. This is the glandular organ which lies behind the stomach and has both an internal and an external secretion. Stone formation anywhere in the body has always been regarded as a diseased condition.

In our opinion, all these stones are formed by the unbalanced, acid, toxin-producing diet that most humans eat; further aggravated by the chemicalized, inorganically mineralized water they drink. Add to this the heavy concentrations of salt most people use, plus the tremendous amount of waxy cholesterol (saturated fats) ingested by the average person, then unhealthful conditions result! Unbalanced diets form toxic poisons which the body cannot metabolize or easily eliminate, so these toxins are formed into stones by the body's chemistry. Practically all drinking water contains the inorganic mineral calcium carbonate. This and other inorganic minerals and toxins play a part in the formation of stones within the body's organs.

Silent, Painless Gallstones
May Suddenly Become Noisy and Painful

"Silent" gallstones are those which remain quietly in the gallbladder and do not produce the acute abdominal pain which is known as gallstone colic. However, these silent stones may at any time – perhaps at an inopportune moment – become raucously "noisy" and extremely painful!

Noisy gallstones may involve not only the gallbladder itself but also the common duct – a vital structure which serves to carry secretions from both the gallbladder and the liver into the intestine. This often happens when the gallbladder contracts and attempts to expel a gallstone. If the stone gets stuck on the way out, there is acute pain and in many cases inflammation of the gallbladder and the common duct.

If the stone blocks the common duct, the liver cannot send its bile into the intestine where it is essential for proper digestion. Then the liver is in trouble! The result is what is known as obstructive jaundice, evidenced by the yellow of the bile which shows up in the skin and in the whites of the eyes.

The color of the skin also betrays the presence of silent gallstones. This was the case with the great Hollywood film actor Tyrone Power, who came to us for health and diet counseling. He looked physically fit, but we could tell from

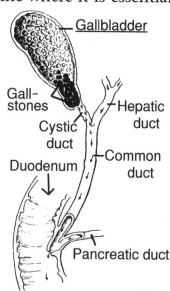

GALLSTONES IN THE GALLBLADDER

Gallstones may be caused by the drinking of water saturated with inorganic minerals and the deadly toxic crystals formed by an unbalanced, unnatural diet. Also, hardened, saturated fats and hydrogenated foods and oils can cause gallbladder problems.

the color of his skin and his eyes that he was suffering with silent gallstones. We pleaded with him to change his unhealthy habits and follow Mother Nature's way, but sadly we could not get him to change! He died way too young! If he had let us put him on a program of liver and gallbladder detoxification – and given up his unbalanced diet, alcohol, salt and ordinary drinking water – that talented, handsome man might still be alive!

We have had many people under our nutritional supervision who had gallstones. The following is an excerpt from the Bragg book, *Apple Cider Vinegar – Miracle Health System.* See back pages for booklist.

Apple Cider Vinegar Combats Gallstones

Before starting the 2 day gallbladder flush, prepare for 1 week by drinking slowly – upon arising, at mid-morning, mid-afternoon and after dinner – 2 tsp. ACV in a 6 ounce glass of organic apple juice; or if diabetic or hypoglycemic dilute with half distilled water. Apple juice is rich in malic acid, potassium, pectins and enzymes that act as solvents to soften and help remove debris (small stones etc.) and cleanse the body. Doctors have new non-surgical methods for removing the difficult, larger stones using sound waves. But it's best to purge the small and medium-sized ones about once or twice a year. These could develop into problems!

53

No food is eaten (only liquids) during the following 2 day gallbladder flush. Fill an 8 ounce glass with one part virgin olive oil (no substitutes) and two parts apple juice (organic is best) and add 1 tsp. ACV. Take this mixture 3 times the first day. *At night, sleep on the right side when on flush, pulling right knee toward chest to open pathway.* On the second day, take the mixture twice. On both days you may drink all the apple juice you desire, but no other liquid, not even water. This treatment is not recommended for diabetics unless supervised by a health professional.

Living under the conditions of modern life, it is important to bear in mind that the preparation and refinement of food products either entirely eliminates or in part destroys the vital elements in the original material.
– U.S. Department of Agriculture

About midmorning on the third day, eat a raw variety salad (nature's broom) of cabbage, carrots, celery, beets, tomatoes, sprouts and lettuce, with generous amounts of ACV and olive oil. If desired, have a bowl of lightly steamed greens, such as kale, collards, chard or other leafy greens. Add ACV and olive oil and a spray of Bragg Liquid Aminos – it gives a delicious flavor to all greens.

We take this miracle cleanser flush at least once a year. Check your bowel movements for tiny, greenish-brown stones. It's amazing what your gallbladder, stomach and colon will flush out!

Kidney Stones

The major cause of most kidney stones is hard, chemicalized water that's saturated heavily with calcium carbonate and other inorganic minerals. Read page 82.

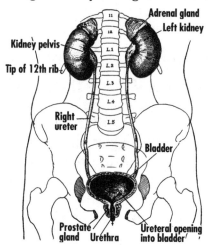

THE URINARY SYSTEM:

THE KIDNEYS, URETERS AND BLADDER. The adrenal glands are shown on top of the kidneys. It is in the urinary system that inorganic minerals and toxic acid crystals may cause kidney and bladder stones. The urinary system must be kept free of these deposits to remain in the healthy elastic condition characteristic of youthfulness.

Beneath our home in the California desert, there is a subterranean river. When wells are sunk into this river several hundred feet below the earth's surface, the water comes out at 180°. It's heavily saturated with calcium carbonate and related minerals, such as magnesium carbonate. This water is not channelled through cast iron or steel pipes because the costly encrustations of these inorganic minerals will soon block the water flow. Copper pipes are the best for hot mineral springs plumbing.

People come from all over the world to bathe in the mineral waters at this spa town. The hot water does have a wonderful curative value. It brings relief to those suffering from arthritis and rheumatism. Most of the hot water pools are kept at a temperature of 104 to 108 degrees. Our body heat is 98.6 degrees. When you submerge your body in water hotter than body temperature, you start an artificial fever and many toxic poisons are eliminated through the 96 million pores of the skin. We all know that a good sweat is refreshing to the body. We always feel lighter after a healthy sweat!

The sad part about coming to the hot water resort, however, is that people are also advised to drink this water that's heavily saturated by inorganic mineral water. And the high concentrations of these inorganic minerals are extremely dangerous! If you put 5 gallons of this mineral water in a pan and let it evaporate, a slab of inorganic minerals will be left.

Don't Drink Inorganic Mineralized Water

Several years ago, a gentleman from New York came to this hot water resort to take the baths. The uninformed owners of the spa told this man to also drink the mineral water, as it would be good for him. We advised him strongly to bathe only – not to drink the water. But he did not heed our advice. During the 6 months he took the baths, he also drank this water that caused his demise! One night the people in the hotel heard him scream out in agonized pain. When they reached him, he was dead. The autopsy showed that he was killed by a large kidney stone which had punctured a major artery.

55

Thousands upon thousands of people all over the world have kidney stones of various shapes and sizes. Sometimes these stones get so troublesome that one kidney must be removed by surgery.

We have visited hot and cold water spas all over the world. The operators of these spas tell people that by drinking and bathing in these waters, various diseases will be cured. We don't believe this! Relief of pain and detoxification of body wastes from bathing in mineral water – yes! But drinking this heavy inorganic mineral water? No! It only causes serious health problems.

> **Our sincere and honest advice to you is:**
> **Don't drink inorganically mineralized water!**

You must always keep in mind that your body cannot assimilate inorganic minerals. You can only assimilate organic minerals which come from a living source (veggies, fruits, grains, etc.).

Dolomite Tablets – Inorganic & Unhealthy

Dolomite tablets are currently sold as a magnesium supplement. These tablets are made from an inorganic limestone source. They contain the same formula that was in the feed purchased many, many years ago for cattle at the Bragg family farm in Virginia. The cattle absolutely refused to eat it! It was finally taken off the market. Similarly, these dolomite tablets cannot be used by humans. **Only organic minerals can be used by the body!** Beware of any pill that is extracted from something advertisers describe as, "The mineral-rich earth!" To use such tablets is not only a waste of money, but also poses a risk to your precious health!

What is Gout?

People are sometimes disturbed when a doctor makes a diagnosis of gout to explain an aching joint, especially in their big toes. Perhaps they remember the old pictures of the British Lord with one leg wrapped up and propped on a chair in front of him, his face bearing an expression of great pain. They may also remember that he arrived at this unhappy state by living high on the hog – gorging himself on a hearty diet of animal flesh, eggs, milk and cheeses, rich sauces and gravies made from meat . . . all washed down with alcohol and chemicalized and inorganically mineralized water.

For more than 85 years, we've seen various versions of the high protein diet come and go. The purveyors of these diets rationalize that because our bodies contain a great deal of protein, we must eat large amounts of it each day to build our bodies and our strength.

Meat protein is heavily saturated with a powerful toxic material called uric acid. Gout occurs as a result of a disturbance in the production, destruction and excretion of uric acid.

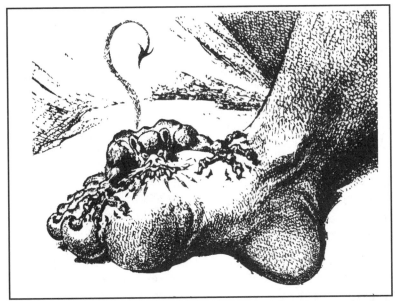

Gout: The Pain is Like a Monster Eating Your Flesh!
Cartoon from an old English drawing.

After the body performs various chemical operations to break down the proteins found in all living cells, this substance – uric acid – is the final end product. A certain amount of it is normally found in the blood, up to about 5 or 6 milligrams per 100 milligrams of blood serum. When this amount is elevated, it increases the likelihood of gout or painful gout-like symptoms.

How do you know if you have this problem? If you have severe, intermittent pain in one of your joints, most often the great toe joint, your doctor may suspect this indicates a special form of joint inflammation (arthritis) known as gouty arthritis or simply gout. As distinguished from chronic arthritis, there is no residual pain or tenderness between the severe, painful attacks.

If the disease goes unchecked, the periods between attacks become shorter and the joint gradually becomes deformed. Toxic crystals formed from uric acid and inorganic minerals in hard drinking water are deposited in joints or bursa, causing the destruction of surrounding tissues. These same deposits are also found in cartilage surrounding bone throughout the body and are called chalk stones or tophi, another characteristic of gout.

The kidneys are often involved in these gouty disturbances. Structures within the kidneys called tubules may be blocked by the crystals deposited by uric acid and inorganic minerals. These toxic crystals are commonly reabsorbed into the body from the kidney tubules, aggravating the trouble. In fact, the most serious complication of gout is kidney damage.

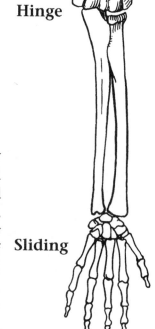

Ball and Socket

It is within the shoulder, elbow, wrist and hand joints that inorganic minerals from salt, hard mineralized water and toxic acid crystals (from the wrong foods, etc.) may form and cripple one or more of these joints, or the legs, hips, back or neck causing pain and restricted movement.

Healthful Ways to Alleviate Gout

Hinge

What can we do about this painful, distressing condition? It's not possible for us to offer cures, but rather to inspire you about healthy lifestyle living so Mother Nature will help you clear up your health problems!

If this misery hits you, the first thing you must do is fast. Fast 1 day a week on 8 glasses of distilled water (cool or warm). You may add 1 to 2 teaspoons equally of organic, raw apple cider vinegar and raw honey. Drinking large amounts of **Sliding** pure, steam-processed distilled water often prevents the formation of kidney stones (which also result from uric acid and drinking water with inorganic minerals).

No man can violate Nature's Laws and escape her penalties! – Julian Johnson

Distilled water is the greatest solvent on earth, the only one that can be taken into the body without damage to the tissues. – Dr. Allen Banik, *The Choice is Clear*

Four Types of Joint Movement

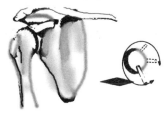

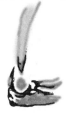

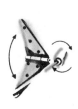

Ball and socket joints – at hips and shoulders permit free movement in all directions.

The vertebrae are saddle joints – moving forward, backward and sideways. One vertebrae moves only slightly on the next, but the whole spinal column is fairly flexible.

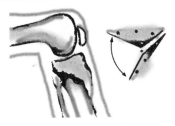

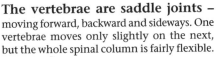

Hinge joints – are like common hinges, permitting backward and forward movement only, like the hinges of a door. Your knees and your fingers are amazing hinge joints.

Pivot joints – permit the bones to rotate at the joint like a key turning in a lock. The elbow is a combination of pivot joint and hinge joint. Thanks to this remarkable joint, one bone of the forearm can rotate about the other.

59

After the distilled water fast, you shouldn't eat foods high in purine. This is a chemical which is called the *parent* of the uric acid substance. The person suffering from gout should not eat any kidneys, liver, sweetbreads, sardines, anchovies or meat extracts. Also avoid alcohol, coffee, sugar, meats, fish, pork, pork products, fowl, peas, beans, nuts, cheese, eggs, milk and dairy products.

Organic Fruits & Vegetables – Nature's Finest

The most protective foods are organic fruits and vegetables. About 60% of your diet should be raw vegetables and fruits and their fresh juices. Properly cooked vegetables, tofu and sunflower or sesame seeds could constitute the protein foods. If a gouty condition still persists then whole grain breads should be eliminated for 6 months. Each week, faithfully take a 24 hour distilled water fast.

Arthritis and Rheumatism

There is a good bit of confusion in the use of the words rheumatism and arthritis. Nowadays, the word rheumatism is used loosely to mean pain and discomfort in and around the joints. In stricter usage, rheumatic conditions include not only those of bone and cartilage, but also of the tendons and tissues surrounding the bones, or their associated connective tissue. We also use the word bursitis when the inflammation is confined to the bursa, a sac containing fluid to prevent friction between joint and tendon.

It is of interest to note that millions of Americans have arthritis problems, making this one of our most common physical complaints. One-tenth are disabled by their arthritis to some degree. All of this indicates that arthritis, which strictly means "inflammation of the joints," is a dreaded condition! It has been estimated that there are more than 50 varieties of this disease. The kind most feared is known as rheumatoid arthritis. All ages may be affected. Even very young children suffer from this misery, which is often deforming.

Rheumatoid arthritis may affect different parts of the body, but the joints are the chief targets. Its onset is characterized by redness, heat and swelling, causing inflammation in one or more of the joints. When a joint is swollen and painful, it is difficult to use and therefore becomes less flexible from lack of use as well as from the misery itself. The muscles also grow smaller or atrophy without exercise. The victim may seem to have large and very sore joints with thin arms and legs.

There is no known cure for rheumatoid arthritis. We have no cures to offer you. Again, all we can offer you is The Bragg Healthy Lifestyle. Only the basic biological functions of your body can help you correct this unhealthy and painful condition.

Distilled water should play a most important part of the treatment for arthritis.
– Dr. Allen Banik, *Your Water and Your Health*

Osteoporosis researchers are confirming in a variety of experiments that the more salt you eat, the more calcium you lose from your body and the more prone you become to debilitating fractures as you age.
– Tufts University Nutrition Letter

POSTURE CHART

	PERFECT	FAIR	POOR
HEAD			
SHOULDERS			
SPINE			
HIPS			
ANKLES			
NECK			
UPPER BACK			
TRUNK			
ABDOMEN			
LOWER BACK			

61

BRAGG POSTURE EXERCISE

Tighten buttocks, suck in stomach muscles, lift up chest, shoulders back, chin up slightly, nose plumb-line to belly button. Swing arms to normalize your posture. Do this often every day to reconstruct your posture to perfection!

Prevention is always preferable to cure!

Health Hints for Aching Muscle and Joints

In order to prevent your important muscles from shriveling and becoming useless, they must be exercised – but only in the correct way. If you don't use your over 640 muscles, you lose them! Besides keeping the muscles from wasting away, the gentle exercises we've suggested for you are designed to preserve the mobility of your joints. Even if it hurts you to exercise the affected areas, you must try to gradually work your muscles loose and flexible and your joints free of the cement-like, toxic chemical crystals. Then the toxins can be dissolved and excreted by your hard working elimination system.

Great relief from pain and swelling may be obtained through heat. Heat relieves the muscle spasms and thus improves the blood flow to both muscles and joints. Usually it is best to apply heat (via a hot bath, heating pad or heat salve – cayenne, etc.) for a little while before exercise. This helps relax the area so you will have an easier time exercising. At the hot mineral spas in California, we see many helpless sufferers of rheumatoid arthritis getting blessed relief from these hot mineral waters. If you can't go to a hot spring for relief, you can take a hot tub soak (massage body while soaking) adding 1 cup of Epsom salts or apple cider vinegar to water.

Bed boards are helpful to prevent the spine from taking on a curve from a soft or sagging mattress. Personally, we sleep on beds without springs – just a thin mattress over a wooden platform. This is a great way to keep the spine supple and strong.

Posture exercises to prevent a curved back and a stooped neck are excellent preventative medicine. In fact, this type of exercise should be done by everyone – even those without any sign of arthritis – to preserve the erectness of youth as long as possible. Walk, stand and sit tall! Make your muscles work to keep you stretched as tall as possible at all times! Most great men of history had good posture and with practice, you can too! Start now! Remember that daily good posture practice will make you more perfect! Reread page 61!

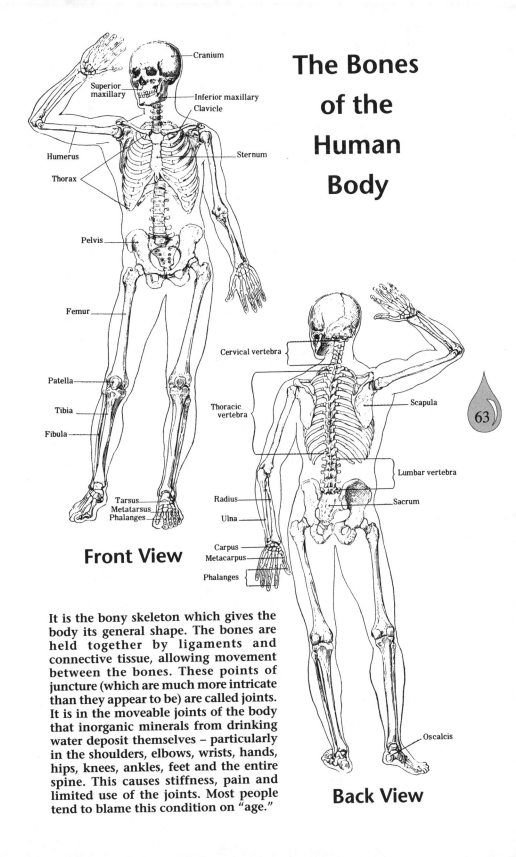

The Bones of the Human Body

Front View

- Cranium
- Superior maxillary
- Inferior maxillary
- Clavicle
- Humerus
- Sternum
- Thorax
- Pelvis
- Femur
- Patella
- Tibia
- Fibula
- Tarsus
- Metatarsus
- Phalanges

Back View

- Cervical vertebra
- Scapula
- Thoracic vertebra
- Lumbar vertebra
- Radius
- Sacrum
- Ulna
- Carpus
- Metacarpus
- Phalanges
- Oscalcis

It is the bony skeleton which gives the body its general shape. The bones are held together by ligaments and connective tissue, allowing movement between the bones. These points of juncture (which are much more intricate than they appear to be) are called joints. It is in the moveable joints of the body that inorganic minerals from drinking water deposit themselves – particularly in the shoulders, elbows, wrists, hands, hips, knees, ankles, feet and the entire spine. This causes stiffness, pain and limited use of the joints. Most people tend to blame this condition on "age."

63

Let us state emphatically that, in our opinion, the misery of arthritis is caused by ingestion of hard water saturated with inorganic minerals and toxins and an unbalanced diet. These factors combined with inactivity can form acid crystals in the moveable joints. Ill health is the result of a combination of unnatural living habits! Every effect must have a cause! There is a reason why things happen in the body. Failure to live Mother Nature's healthy lifestyle is the cause of human miseries.

Posture Silhouettes

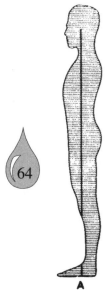 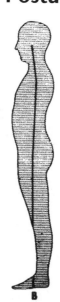 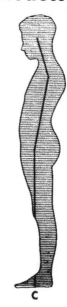 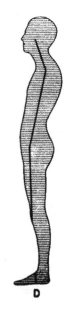

A. Good: head, trunk and thigh are in a straight line; chest is held forward and high; the abdomen is flat and the back curves normally.

B. Fair: the head is held forward and abdomen is prominent with an exaggerated curve in upper back; slightly hollowed back.

C. Poor: a relaxed and fatigued posture; head is forward and abdomen is relaxed; the shoulder blades are prominent; hollowed back.

D. Very Poor: head pushed forward; very exaggerated curve in upper back; the abdomen relaxed; flat–sloping chest; hollowed back.

Don't Let Your Brain Turn to Stone

Our neighbor, James K., is 65 years old. You will note that we said 65 years old, unfortunately not 65 years young. Jim will be forced to retire from his position as an executive in a large company in a few months. This is becoming an enforced company rule across America!

Nine men in ten are suicides. – Ben Franklin

Why do so many large corporations require all employees to retire at age 65? The main reason is that by age 65, most people have hardening of the arteries of the brain. The brain has lost much of its blood supply and is not getting the life-giving oxygen that it needs to keep it healthy, sharp, creative, wide-awake and positive.

Remember that many of the capillaries supplying the brain are as small as a human hair. Years of drinking chemicalized, inorganic mineral water and years of eating a highly unbalanced diet heavy in salt has created masses of toxic acid crystals. These crystals harden the arteries, veins and capillaries that must supply the brain with the needed blood for full brain power.

The Nervous System is the Communication Network of the Body

There is a definite link between physical vigor and mental vigor. It all comes down to the fact that we must have a sound mind in a healthy body.

People actually build rock formations in the blood vessels supplying blood to their brains, just as the great rock formations are made in limestone caverns. You can see how these great columns of stalactites and stalagmites are formed, one drop at a time by inorganic mineral water. The brain does not turn into stone in a few years. But year after year of ingesting inorganic mineral water and toxic foods will slowly build these rock formations in your brain and throughout your body!

The nervous system, which is made up of the brain and nerves, is the communication system of the body. Note that the nerves vary considerably in diameter and length.

Let nature be your teacher. – William Wordsworth

Doomed to the Human Scrap Pile

Most big corporations are less likely to hire someone who is 50 years of age. They know from actual experience that there is considerable brain deterioration and brain slow down in the majority of people over 50.

It all boils down to simple physics (basic physiological facts). You have small blood vessels leading to your brain. The way the average person avoids exercise, eats junk and drinks hard water invites degenerative changes in these blood vessels throughout the body and especially in the brain. The longer the average person lives in this manner, the more body degeneration takes place!

Many senior citizens will admit that their mental faculties seem to be slipping. They will tell you how poor their memory has become and how they cannot always recall names and events. A brain turning to stone does not have the capacity to be wide awake and sharp! As this condition gets worse, we call it senility. In time, the brain solidifies to a point where it remembers nothing. This is called living in deep senility or Alzheimer's disease. Or is it a living death?

66

How the Brain Functions

Did you ever stop to consider what makes you think? Inside the protective covering of the bony skull is a mass of what we call "gray matter." Gray matter is tissue composed of millions of nerve cells "woven" together – enabling what we see, hear, taste and touch to give us an awareness of our status on this earth.

Using our gray matter, we also think, know, remember, judge and believe. It was named gray matter because it is largely pinkish-gray in color. The brain also has a white part. Our behavior and emotions are controlled by this mass of tissue. We now know that the secretions of the endocrine glands also affect the stream of communications, which in turn alters the brain cells.

This structure, the brain, is an incredibly complex electrochemical organ, as individual to each of us as are fingerprints. It is the miracle of life – a miracle which

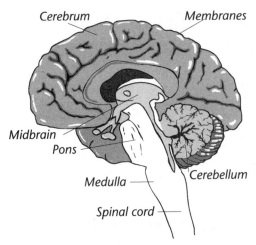

Cerebrum   Membranes

Midbrain
Pons
Medulla
Cerebellum
Spinal cord

ADULT BRAIN

The adult brain, the human computer, weighs about 3 pounds, but it powerfully directs all of your thoughts, feelings and actions.

gives us joy and sorrow, philosophy and politics, understanding and reasoning power, will power and the ability to have feelings. Philosophers have called it "man's unconquerable mind." As we see what has been developed by it from one century to another, we can almost call the adjective "unconquerable" a factual one.

As the average person's brain slowly turns to stone, much of their birthright of keen awareness is lost. Eyesight starts to go as cataracts develop (a stony film formation over the eyes). Hearing becomes impaired because the arteries leading to the ears become corroded with inorganic mineral encrustations. These are all diseases of degeneration, which most people blame on the passing years, not on how badly they have lived.

This gray matter we call the brain must have oxygenated blood or it degenerates! All living cells of the body must have oxygen in large quantities to survive. Senility is caused by the oxygen starvation of the brain.

To possess an ageless and unconquerable mind, we must constantly provide it with a free flow of life-giving, oxygen-rich, red blood. That is the reason the supply pipes leading to the brain must not be blocked by encrusted inorganic minerals. If you wish to maintain or regain a strong brain, use only steam-produced distilled water and fresh fruit and vegetable juices as your drinks. Keep far away from city, well and tap waters, alcohol, tea, coffee, cola and soft drinks.

The Brain Needs High Quality Nutrition

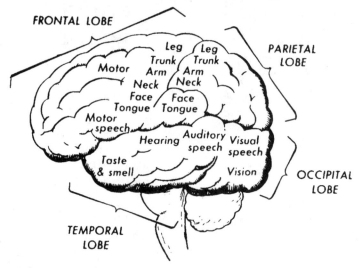

FRONTAL LOBE

PARIETAL LOBE

Leg / Leg
Trunk / Trunk
Motor / Arm / Arm
Neck / Neck
Face / Face
Tongue / Tongue
Motor
speech
Hearing / Auditory / Visual
speech / speech
Taste
& smell
Vision

OCCIPITAL LOBE

TEMPORAL LOBE

Above shows control areas – everything you do – including seeing, hearing, speaking, breathing or moving – is controlled by a part of your brain.

68

The brain must be adequately nourished in order to function properly. No other part of the body fails more quickly from lack of good nutrition. Upon what does this marvelous structure feed? It needs foods rich in enzymes. Organic raw fruits and vegetables and their fresh juices provide excellent nourishment. Soy beans, which are exceptionally rich in lecithin, should be eaten several times weekly. Lecithin in powdered, liquid, capsule, tablet or granulated form can also be purchased at your health food store. Raw, unsalted sunflower, sesame and pumpkin seeds are all healthful brain foods.

Neuron

The entire nervous system is made of individual cells called neurons. Every neuron has 3 main parts: the cell body, the dendrite, and the axon.

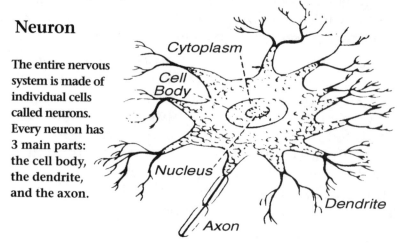

Cytoplasm

Cell Body

Nucleus

Dendrite

Axon

Organic Minerals are Essential to Life

The brain needs phosphorus. Organic phosphorus is found in beans of all kinds including: pinto, garbanzo and dried lima beans and lentils. Other phosphorus rich sources are: 100% whole grains, brown rice, almonds, peanuts and walnuts. Lean meats, egg yolks and natural, unprocessed cheeses also contain organic phosphorus.

All the organic minerals are needed to keep the body strong, youthful and healthy. They are essential factors in digestion and assimilation, constituting important ingredients of the digestive juices and regulating the osmotic exchange between lymph and blood cells. In short, organic minerals are indispensable to the proper physiological functioning of all the systems of the body.

Organic Minerals Make the Man!

It is estimated that an average man weighing 150 pounds is composed of the following:

90 lbs. oxygen
36 lbs. carbon
14 lbs. hydrogen
3 lbs. 8 oz. nitrogen
3 lbs. 12 oz. calcium
1 lb. 4 oz. phosphorus
32 oz. sulphur
3 oz. potassium
22 oz. sodium
12 oz. magnesium
4 oz. silicon
6 oz. iron

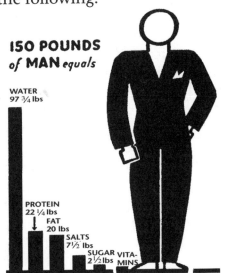

150 POUNDS *of* **MAN** *equals*

WATER 97 ¾ lbs
PROTEIN 22 ¼ lbs
FAT 20 lbs
SALTS 7½ lbs
SUGAR 2½ lbs
VITA-MINS

Trace Elements

Our bodies are also made up of trace amounts of these other important elements: manganese, zinc, neon, iodine, copper, lithium, cobalt, helium, etc.

It is a mistake to think that the more a man eats, the stronger he will become.

Formula for Creating a Human Being

According to B. A. Howard – in his book *The Proper Study of Mankind* – the human body contains:

- Enough water to fill a 10 gallon barrel.
- Enough fat to make 7 bars of soap.
- Enough carbon for 9,000 lead pencils.
- Enough phosphorus for 2,200 match-heads.
- Just enough iron for 1 medium-size nail.
- Enough calcium (lime) to whitewash a chicken coop.
- And microscopic amounts of such trace elements as cobalt, iodine, zinc, copper, molybdenum, titanium, beryllium, etc.

Take these ingredients; combine them in the right proportions and in the right way; and the result, apparently, is the creation of a man.

The Body is Composed of Organic Minerals

Remember that these are **ALL ORGANIC** – not inorganic – chemicals and minerals. There is a sharp line of demarcation between the two! Although the chemical analysis is the same whether found in air, earth, plant or animal – it is only through the life processes of the plant whereby the constituents of air and soil become vitalized and useful to the human body. It is this property of vitality alone which distinguishes, for example, the atom of iron in the red corpuscles of the blood from that of inorganic iron or preparations made from inorganic iron. You could suck on an iron nail for years and never extract any organic iron for building your blood. When you eat blackberries, you are getting organic iron that can be used by the blood. The arrangement of atoms that form a molecule of the iron nail is the same as that of the organic iron in the blackberry. Only by the great natural miracle force of photosynthesis does the living plant convert the inert inorganic minerals into the organic minerals which we can use for keeping ourselves alive and healthy!

Nature never deceives us; it is always we who deceive ourselves. – Rousseau

Sometimes the minerals of the body are referred to as "mineral salts." This misleading terminology has given the public the wrong idea that this term "salt" refers to common table salt, or inorganic sodium chloride. Most people mistakenly consider added salt an indispensable adjunct to almost all foods and part of a healthy diet.

The fact cannot be over-emphasized that there is a vital change going on in all the minerals as they are absorbed into the structure of the plant. On the other hand, chemical analysis or separation of the minerals means destruction of the living tissues. But of course, the chemist will find in the minerals of the "ash" those same properties that are present in the minerals of the soil. But that subtle, imponderable force – vital electricity (the life force of plants) – has escaped him. It cannot be isolated by the laboratory processes of condensation or extraction. We must learn to recognize the mineral elements of the body as really being "organic" components – internal parts of the living body and subject to the same vital changes, life and death that affect the organism.

The organic calcium in the skeleton, the organic iron contained in the red corpuscles and the organic sodium and potassium found in the blood serum are biologically organized. They have a certain duration of life during which they have vital functions to perform. Sooner or later these molecules will lose their electromagnetic tension, according to the degree of their physiological activity. In other words, they have served their purpose and must be supplanted by fresh organic minerals. That is the reason that 60% –70% of your diet should be fresh, living raw fruits and vegetables. These are the great suppliers of the imponderable life force – vital electricity.

The Alkaline or Base-Forming Minerals

The alkaline minerals – which are so important in the performance of the physiological functions of the body – are iron, sodium, calcium, magnesium, potassium and manganese. These are the eliminators of toxic waste poisons, the real immunizers of body. They are essential to the formation of the digestive juices and the secretions of the ductless glands (these hormones probably regulate nearly all the vital processes of the body).

Iron is necessary for the formation of red blood corpuscles and acts as the oxygen carrier of the system. Elimination of carbon dioxide depends largely upon organic sodium, which is the chief constituent of the blood and lymph. Calcium, combined with magnesium, phosphorus and silicon, makes up more than half of the bony structure of the body and imparts strength to all tissues. It also serves as a neutralizer and eliminator of toxic acids. Remember, whenever we refer to minerals in the body, we are speaking of **organic** minerals.

The Lower Respiratory System

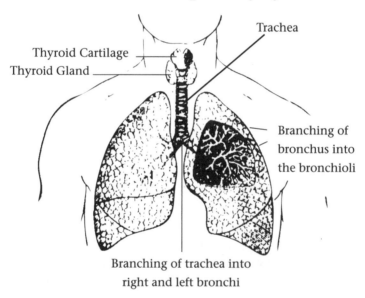

Thyroid Cartilage

Thyroid Gland

Trachea

Branching of bronchus into the bronchioli

Branching of trachea into right and left bronchi

This is where inorganic minerals and toxic acid crystals that can cause serious trouble in the respiratory system deposit themselves, slowing down the needed supply of life-giving oxygen.

Inorganic Water Turns People to Stone

When my dad was a small boy, his father took him and the other children of the family from their Virginia home to Washington, D.C., to see the P.T. Barnum Circus. To a boy from a farm this was a great event! After seeing the big circus show in the big tent, they visited the "Side

Show" tent where all the unusual, so-called "freaks" were exhibited. There were fat men and women – some weighing as much as 600 pounds – dwarfs, giants, the bearded lady, the monkey man and others.

But the one that most fascinated my dad was the lady who had turned to stone. There was a woman on a bed who was so full of arthritis and acid crystals that she had no feeling left in her petrified body. She lay helpless and rigid. She could move only her eyes. This lady suffered from complete ankylosis – meaning that no joint in her entire body could make a simple movement. All the nerve tissue in her body was paralyzed and dead – they could actually drive nails into her body! The man who explained these "freaks" said that this lady was born in Hot Springs, Arkansas, which explained it, as my father later discovered.

Stone Lady Mystery Solved

The lady who had turned to stone was a complete mystery to my father as a child. But not today! The water in Hot Springs is some of the hardest water in the United States. We have seen chemical analyses of it and the concentrations of calcium carbonate, potassium carbonate and magnesium carbonate are very, very high. That poor lady in the side show was a victim of this inorganic water. Her vital organs were not strong enough to flush those inorganic minerals out of her body, so they deposited themselves in her joints. This was an unusual and extreme case, of course. But we've seen many, many cases of arthritics who were complete cripples, absolutely helpless. There are more than 20 million people young and old living in the United States today who suffer from arthritis to some degree.

Nothing can bring you peace but yourself. – Ralph Waldo Emerson

Learn now what and how great benefits a temperate diet will bring along with it. In the first place, you will enjoy good health. – Horace, 65 B.C.

God sends the food. Man, by refining and processing the food, destroys its nutritional value. Eat only God's natural food. – Patricia Bragg

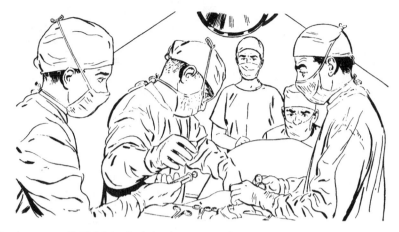

There are over 8,000 hospitals in the U.S.A. where surgery goes on around the clock. Many people undergo orthopedic surgery to have joint replacements and painful bone spurs removed, as well as bladder stones, kidney stones and gallstones. Will you be next?

Bone Spurs and Moveable Joint Calcification

74

Every day large numbers of people go into surgery to have joint replacements or to have painful, crippling bone spurs removed or to have calcified deposits removed from their moveable joints. These bone spurs and calcified formations are insoluble deposits that get into the tissues after consumption of water loaded with inorganic minerals, salt and uric acid, plus deposited toxic acid crystals from an incorrect diet high in acid. Meat, potatoes, refined flour, white bread, coffee, tea and sugary desserts are all high in acid content. This unfortunately is the dead-food diet that most people eat. This diet, combined with hard water, is why there are so many troubles resulting from acid deposits that create bone spurs and painful crystallized joints, etc.

Deposits of Inorganic Minerals and Toxic Acid Crystals in the Heel of the Foot, Causing Great Pain!

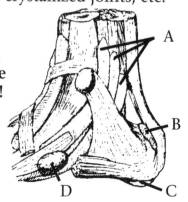

A. Inorganic minerals deposited under the tendons.

B. Under the Achilles tendon.

C. Under the heel.

D. Under the middle foot.

Do It Yourself Calcification Test

Take this test to discover just how calcified your joints have become:

Stand erect, hands hanging loosely at your sides. Now lower your head to your chest and start a slow rolling movement, around and around. Many people can feel the inorganic calcification grating as they roll their heads. This shows that there has been a definite infiltration of insoluble minerals and toxic acid crystals into the head of the atlas, the bone at the top of the spine upon which the skull rests.

Also test the moveable joints of your body. Do you have stiffness? How limber is your spine? Can you raise your hands over your head and bend forward with your knees locked to touch the floor with your fingertips? Are you limber enough to place the palms of your hands on the floor as you keep your knees stiff?

Stand with your back to a wall. Move forward about 2 feet, then bend backward and "walk" down the wall with your hands. How far can you go?

How high can you kick? Do you have cracking in your knees when you do a leg squat? How flexible are your feet? Do you walk with a spring in your step? Do you have a feeling of suppleness and flexibility in your body? Do you walk and dance with grace, or do you walk on calcified encrustations that cause you misery and pain? Is your body flexible and pain free?

Don't say your stiffness is due to your age! That is just so much rubbish! You can keep your body youthful and flexible with proper care!

Perfection consists not in doing extraordinary things, but in doing ordinary things extraordinarily well. Neglect nothing; the most trivial action may be performed with joy. – Angelique Arnauld

The USA per capita daily home consumption of water – kitchen, bathing, laundry, etc. – is 60 gallons per person or 14 billion gallons daily.

It is never too late to begin getting into shape, but it does take daily, sometimes painful perseverance. – Thomas K. Cureton

Organic Calcium is Important for a Fit Heart

Most people correctly associate calcium with the teeth and bones, which is true since a deficiency of this important mineral causes serious damage. Calcium is very important for the nerves of the body; many people suffer from leg cramps due to a calcium deficiency.

Calcium also plays a very important role in the functioning of the human heart. It is a natural constituent of the material that causes the blood to clot. If we did not have calcium in our bloodstream, we could prick a finger with a needle and bleed to death!

Every few minutes the heart is bathed by the calcium of the body chemistry. It is important to the very life of the heart's activity. Being the most powerful muscle in the entire body, the heart requires adequate calcium for its normal functioning. Now consider the shocking fact that *85% of the American people are deficient in calcium!*

76

New Information Regarding Calcium Requirements for Healthy Bodies

The National Academy of Sciences states that the average consumption of 700-800 milligrams of calcium per day by American adults is not sufficient enough to prevent the bone loss and fractures that result from osteoporosis. The new recommended Dietary Allowances (RDAs), updated in 1998, are now called Dietary Reference Intakes (DRIs). Until now, 800 milligrams of calcium was the daily target for adults. According to the new DRI for calcium, adults aged 19 through 50 should strive to get 1,000 milligrams of calcium daily and those over 50 should aim for 1,200 milligrams. These new guidelines also set higher maximum limits for calcium intake to 2,500 milligrams per day.

Every day the average heart, your best friend, beats 10,000 times and pumps 2,000 gallons of blood for nourishing your body. In 70 years that adds up to more than 360 million (faithful) heartbeats. Please be good to your heart and live The Bragg Healthy Lifestyle for a long happy, healthy life! Here's to Genesis 6:3 for you. – Patricia Bragg

Calcified Toenails and Fingernails

Inorganic minerals, salt and toxic acid crystals can deform the toe and fingernails. We've both seen toes and fingers that were made into monstrosities by calcified joints and nails. Big, thick toenails that are hard as cement and that no pair of scissors or clippers can cut – they have to be filed down with a rugged file – and can often deform the feet, make walking extremely painful and are also a hideous sight.

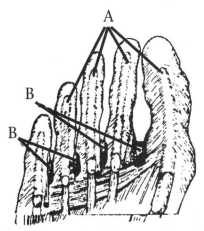

Inorganic Mineral Deposits Between the Bones of the Toes (A,B) Cause Stiffness in the Feet.

Inorganic Deposits Cause Bad Posture

Inorganic minerals and toxic acid crystals are a major cause of poor posture, which brings on all sorts of disturbances by throwing the vital organs out of place, unduly straining some muscles while weakening others, impairing circulation, breathing and elimination.

Just stand on any busy city corner and watch the people go by. What a miserable sight most of them present – people whose feet are so loaded with inorganic calcification that they simply lift their feet up and put them down! The spring's absolutely gone from their step.

GOOD AND BAD WAYS TO:

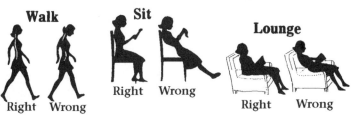

Walk — Right Wrong
Sit — Right Wrong
Lounge — Right Wrong

Many people walk like ducks with their toes pointing outward. Others are stooped and bent out of shape. Some walk with no knee action. You see many whose steps are unsteady because their joints are so cemented and others who are so out of balance that they sway from side to side as they hobble along. Their heads are carried too far forward, throwing their bodies off balance. Watch them as they try to sit down. They simply slump into the chair, giving their lower back a shock.

Water – The Curse of an Aching Back

By the time they reach 40, millions of Americans are plagued by lower back pains. When they bend over it is absolute agony! Their whole lower spine is becoming fossilized and cemented with inorganic calcification.

By the time people are 40, they've worn out much of the cartilage that acts as a cushion to the spinal bones. This is a painful condition which only gets progressively worse on a constant diet of chemicalized and mineralized water. Plus, most suffer from extreme dehydration that, combined with their unhealthy acid crystal-forming diet, adds to their overall joint and health problems.

Proper Walking Posture

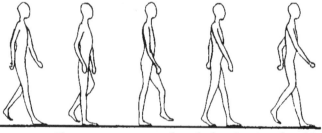

Proper walking posture. Always prepare a new base before leaving the old.

Proper Lifting Posture

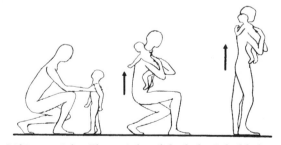

Lifting weight. The weight of the baby is held close to the center of gravity, directly above the pushing force.

The Parade of the "Living Dead"

Just remember that chemically, physically and mentally we are what we eat and drink. Because most humans are ignorant about what to put into their bodies, very few escape being one of the "living dead." So many people, after their 20s, do not know what healthy, vibrant, youthful living is! They drag themselves through life, relying on some kind of medication to keep them going. They need a "pep" pill to keep them going during the day and a sleeping pill to put them to sleep at night.

Check Your Mattress

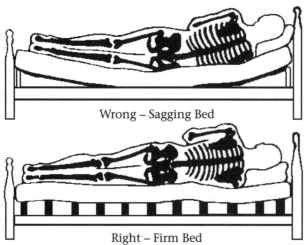

Wrong – Sagging Bed

Right – Firm Bed

During sleep, you recharge the battery you ran down slowly during the day. The right kind of mattress is important. It's better to sleep ON a mattress; not IN it.

Mankind is Sick and Growing Sicker!

Throughout the whole of recorded history, man has suffered with a variety of miseries, a great many of which can be directly traced to hard, inorganic mineral water. In a Milwaukee museum, we saw the backbones (spines) of American Indians who lived in Wisconsin over a thousand years ago, all with calcification that showed they were victims of arthritis. These Indians drank the Lake Michigan water, which is heavily saturated with inorganic calcium carbonate and other inorganic minerals. Their spring and river waters were no better.

One thing they did not have to worry about, however, was the harmful chlorination and fluoridation of their drinking water which would have added more poisons to their already burdened bodies. Even the mummies of ancient Egypt, some over 2,500 years old, show the ravages of arthritis and other diseases due to drinking Nile River water, which is heavily saturated with inorganic minerals.

You can see, even those ancient people, living under the most natural conditions, suffered and died long before their time! Inorganically mineralized water truly is the universal drink of disease and premature death!

Every time a person turns on the water faucet and drinks water that has been chemicalized with chlorine or is saturated with calcium carbonate and other inorganic minerals, he is jeopardizing his health, his mind and his life!

Disfiguring Broken Capillaries

Among the many manifestations of inorganic calcification are broken facial capillaries. Study people's faces. Look closely at the cheek, around the nose and on the chin, where you will often see the smallest blood vessels, slender as hairs, showing near the surface of the skin. When these tiny capillaries become encrusted with inorganic minerals, they expand in size and often rupture, making purplish or reddish blotches. Blocked by inorganic minerals and no longer able to handle the circulation of the blood, except perhaps to a small degree, these broken capillaries not only give the face a grotesque appearance but are often quite painful.

Cold Feet and Cold Hands

Many people of all ages suffer from poor circulation, in most cases due to or aggravated by inorganic mineral encrustations in the arteries, veins and capillaries that constitute the blood circulatory system.

According to the ancient Hindu scriptures, the proper amount of food is half of what can be conveniently eaten.

We have frequently shaken hands with people whose hands were ice cold even on the warmest days. Many people also suffer from extremely cold feet, especially in cool weather. By age 60, most people have patches of small blue, broken and expanded veins around their feet and ankles, giving their legs an appearance of blackness or dirtiness, even just after a bath.

Poor circulation is first and most critically noticeable in the hands and feet because the blood has farther to go from the heart to reach these extremities. When the pipes of the body become clogged and obstructed, the blood has difficulty in getting through. Instead of coursing through the capillaries of the hands and feet in a warm, healthy stream, it trickles through – barely able to bring nourishment, much less any warmth.

The entire body, of course, is affected when the pipes of the circulatory system are clogged. People with poor circulation find it difficult to keep warm in cold or even cool weather. Their homes are overheated and they must bundle up in sweaters, coats and other bulky clothing when they go outside.

Every sick person usually has a sluggish circulatory system that is operating on a very low level – chiefly due to plugged-up pipes. Remember that the main source of these encrustations is drinking water saturated with inorganic minerals. Those who drink distilled water and the juices of fruits and vegetables are helping to keep their circulatory systems clean and more healthy.

CLOGGED PIPES

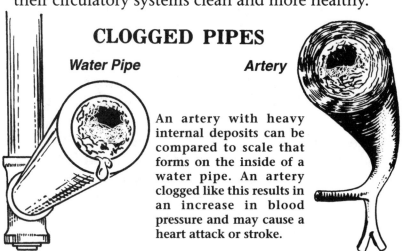

Water Pipe

Artery

An artery with heavy internal deposits can be compared to scale that forms on the inside of a water pipe. An artery clogged like this results in an increase in blood pressure and may cause a heart attack or stroke.

Stop Kidney Stones Cold*

It is hard to believe that something as small as a kidney stone could cause such severe pain. Most people who have suffered through such an episode are highly motivated to do anything necessary to avoid another attack. By making certain lifestyle and diet changes, kidney stone attacks can be prevented.

Kidney stones are composed of waste products – things the body doesn't use or need. Normally these wastes are eliminated through your kidneys in urine, but when there is too much waste or not enough fluid to flush it out, it all comes together to form a stone. The elimination of these stones is what causes the excruciating pain.

By drinking 8 or more 8 oz. glasses of pure distilled water daily and eating less of the foods that form crystals you can prevent the recurrence of kidney stones. Fluids are the single most important ingredient in the prevention of stones. It is important to not get dehydrated and to stay away from hard, artificially softened or mineral waters. Salt, alcohol, inorganic calcium, animal proteins and oxalates are diet "dangers" in the stone-forming process.

Calcium is the most abundant mineral found in kidney stones and calcium stone-formers generally have high urinary calcium. But a low-calcium diet is not recommended because of bone loss and osteoporosis. Stone-formers are urged to consume the equivalent of 800 to 1,000 milligrams (mg) of dietary calcium.

Salt (inorganic sodium) in the diet affects the way your kidneys handle calcium, causing excretion of more calcium, thus increasing your risk of forming stones. Excess amounts of Vitamin C and D can cause stone formation. Alcohol inhibits the ability of the kidneys to excrete uric acid.

Kidney stones can be prevented by following The Bragg Healthy Lifestyle and drinking pure distilled water. Kidney stones really are "what you eat and drink!"

---

*Excerpted from No More Kidney Stones! by John S. Rodman, Cynthia Seidman, and Rory Jones.

Exercises for Healthy Feet

Do these simple exercises daily to help keep feet in good healthy condition and improve circulation:

1. Raise the weight of the body on the toes.
2. Grasp with your toes, pick up a pencil, etc.
3. Sitting in chair with legs outstretched, curl toes up and then stretch toes down and under.
4. In same position as #3, rotate feet clockwise several times. Then repeat, rotating feet counterclockwise.
5. Sit on floor with soles of feet together; pull the heels and toes alternately apart.
6. Stand with your feet parallel, 5 to 6 inches apart; bend the knees and turn them outward while keeping the feet flat on the floor and bend down slightly.
7. Walk barefooted on soft grass or sand anytime the opportunity arises. Your feet love contact with the earth, plus the exercise and the increase in circulation all help to build healthy feet.
8. As soon as you come into the house you should remove your shoes – remember, barefooted is best!
9. Give yourself or your partner first a vinegar foot soak (2 tbsp ACV in hot water) then a foot massage while watching TV or listening to music – rotate, work, kneed and apply pressure to soles for healing delights.

83

Not only do foot soaks and massages help tired and aching feet, but elevating the feet by putting them up on wall, back of couch or by holding them in air for ten minutes helps reduce congestion and varicose veins. Resting the feet is as important as resting the body.

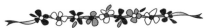

For more foot and vinegar treatments read the Bragg book
Apple Cider Vinegar – Miracle Health System. *See back pages.*

The healing power of massage reduces stress, back and foot pain, and helps fight depression, fatigue, anxiety and helps save lives. – Patricia Bragg

A wise man should consider that health is the greatest of human blessings!
– Hippocrates, Father of Medicine, 400 B.C.

Destiny is not a matter of chance; it is a matter of choice. It is not a thing to be waited for, it is a thing to be achieved. – William Jennings Bryan

Head Noises and Ringing in Ears

Many humans are plagued by head noises, ringing and pounding in the ears. Every waking hour is torture as these head noises wear down their nerve energy. Even in sleep, they have bad dreams about these noises. These head noises may torment them 24 hours a day.

The blood vessels – arteries, veins and capillaries – in the delicate canals of the ears have become hardened and obstructed by inorganic mineral encrustations from hard water, as well as uric acid and deposits of toxic acid crystals from unbalanced diets. This condition produces the head noises – buzzing sounds, ringing and pounding in the ears.

In time, the blood vessels of the ears become so clogged that the person gradually goes deaf. Thousands of people go deaf every year for this reason alone! For a time, they can get some relief from a hearing aid, but many will eventually lose their hearing completely.

84

Human Ear

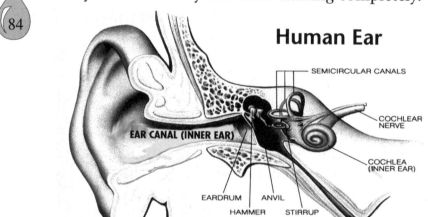

SEMICIRCULAR CANALS

COCHLEAR NERVE

EAR CANAL (INNER EAR)

COCHLEA (INNER EAR)

EARDRUM   ANVIL

HAMMER   STIRRUP

MIDDLE EAR

EUSTACHIAN TUBE

Inorganic Minerals and Toxins Affect the Eyes

Inorganic minerals, toxic poisons and uric acid also have a degenerative effect upon the eyes. Your eyes are among your most important physical possessions. They are often described as the mirror of the soul, the mind and the thoughts. It is true that your eyes often reveal your innermost feelings. Their lustre changes because of psychological influences – such as fear, love, hatred – and because of physical malfunctions. Without your eyes, you would live in total darkness. Many people do!

Sectional View of Right Eyeball

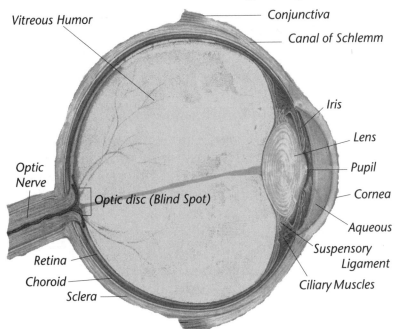

Vitreous Humor — *Conjunctiva*

Canal of Schlemm

Iris

Lens

Optic Nerve

Pupil

Optic disc (Blind Spot)

Cornea

Aqueous

Suspensory Ligament

Retina

Choroid

Ciliary Muscles

Sclera

Now let us examine this miracle mechanism – the eye. The eyeball is an almost spherical body with a mirror at the back portion, the retina. The body of the eye is made up of a transparent jelly-like substance. From the back of the eye runs the optic sensory nerve. This is a head nerve, a major part of the central nervous system.

In the front of the eye there is a crystalline biconvex lens, which is more convex behind the cornea. The white portion of the eye is a fibrous material surrounding the central, colored part – varying in shades of brown, blue, hazel or gray – known as the iris. The iris serves as a photosensitive diaphragm, controlling the amount of light which enters the pupil, the black spot in the center of the eye. When the outside light is bright, the muscles of the iris contract the pupil to a small dot. When the outside light grows dimmer, the pupil expands proportionally to admit more light.

Natural Foods Help Protect Your Eyes

As you see, the eye is a delicate mechanism. All the blood vessels which bring needed nourishment and oxygen to the eye are very tiny capillaries. Year after year, most people drink chemicalized and inorganically mineralized water and absorb the toxic uric acids from their daily food. Just as in the limestone caverns the stalactites and stalagmites are formed drop by drop, so,

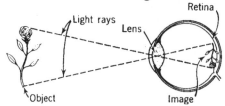

The human eye is very much like a camera. Light rays enter the eye, cross in the lens and focus on the retina.

drop by drop, the blood deposits inorganic minerals and toxic acids into the tiny blood capillaries of the eyes. Encrustations are eventually formed in these delicate capillaries. Glasses are prescribed. After a time stronger glasses are necessary. Then the vision starts to fail and, in some instances, a person is left in total darkness.

Many people panic when they start losing their precious vision. They try treatments of all kinds and descriptions; some have operations, but their sight gradually fades away. Remember that there are three vicious enemies of healthy eyes: inorganic mineral water, toxic poisons from acid-forming foods and uric acid from a diet too heavy in animal proteins.

Build Clean, Healthy Blood

The blood holds the key to our health, vitality and our youthfulness – and our very life! **Keep the blood free from inorganic minerals and toxic acids!**

Every 90 days we build a brand new bloodstream. We can live and regain health using a reversal program being careful of the kind of water we drink and the kind of foods we eat. Starting today you can discard the materials which create an unhealthy bloodstream and start building one that is going to give you a painless, tireless and ageless body! It's all in your hands!

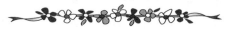

Health and cheerfulness mutually beget each other. – Joseph Addison

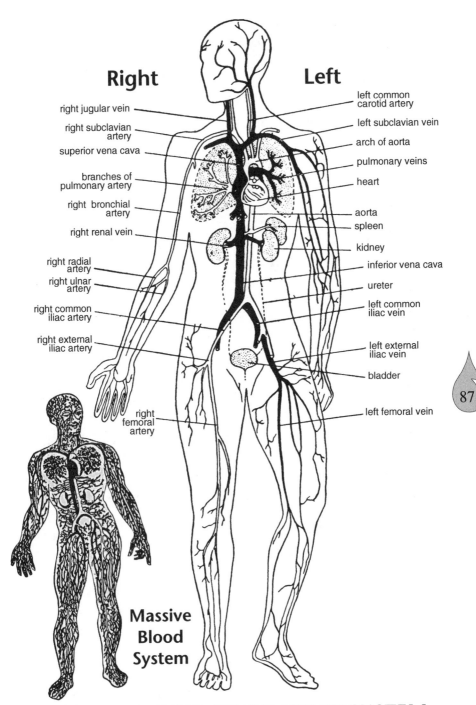

Right

Left

right jugular vein

right subclavian artery

superior vena cava

branches of pulmonary artery

right bronchial artery

right renal vein

right radial artery

right ulnar artery

right common iliac artery

right external iliac artery

right femoral artery

left common carotid artery

left subclavian vein

arch of aorta

pulmonary veins

heart

aorta

spleen

kidney

inferior vena cava

ureter

left common iliac vein

left external iliac vein

bladder

left femoral vein

87

**Massive
Blood
System**

DIAGRAM OF THE CIRCULATORY SYSTEM

For the sake of clarity most blood vessels are not shown
on the larger art. We show only some of the arteries and
veins. The smaller art shows the entire body blood system.

Using the knowledge offered in this book, you can start becoming more youthful as you live longer. You must be the absolute master of what goes into your body in the way of food and drink. Flesh is dumb! Your body will accept almost all foods. That is the reason you must read this book several times and start **living The Bragg Healthy Lifestyle for building clean healthy blood**!

Of course, we all know what blood looks like . . . a somewhat thickish red fluid that we see whenever the skin is even slightly broken. These tiny oozings of blood come from very tiny blood vessels which supply the skin all over the body. Blood, your 'River of Life', is the fluid which carries oxygen and nutrition to all the cells of the body and tries to remove any poisonous substances. The trouble is that the average person is pouring inorganic minerals and toxic poisons into the body so fast that the blood finds it impossible to purify itself, much less the body. Nothing could be more important than this "life blood" of ours. If we do not get enough oxygen and nutrition and if toxic materials are not removed regularly, they will stockpile and we will die.

And that, we're sorry to say, is why most die long before their time. People do not take the time to learn how to get more oxygen into the body; they do not take time or interest in good nutrition. Death comes from accumulated toxins that actually poison and clog up the bloodstream, brain, organs and nerves. The heavy concentrations of inorganic minerals, salt, fat and toxic poisons which are a burden to the body are the vicious killers! Years are not your enemies! It's what you put into your body that does the terrible damage to your health and erodes your future longevity!

Many people go through life committing partial suicide – destroying their health, youth, talents, energies and creative qualities. Indeed, to learn how to be good to oneself is harder than learning how to be good to others. – Joshua Liebman

Eat not for the pleasure thou mayest find therein; eat to increase thy strength, eat to preserve the life thou hast received from Heaven. – Confucius

Chapter 5

Organic Minerals

Iron, the Oxygen Carrier of the Blood

Organic iron is indispensable to the formation of chlorophyll and hemoglobin. Because of its great affinity for oxygen, iron plays an important part in the organic world. It has a very close relationship to the fundamental processes of biological transformation of matter known as metabolism.

The plant or tree takes the inorganic iron from the soil. It carries the iron to the leaves where it takes part in the formation of the chlorophyll granules (the green coloring matter of plants). The amount of organic iron and chlorophyll varies in different parts of the plant. For instance, the green outer leaves of cabbage contain four times as much iron as the inner leaves.

89

How Plants Do Their Miracle Work

In order to carry out their life processes, every organism is equipped with structures enabling it to use the materials in its environment to satisfy its needs. Animals, with their power of locomotion, are able to hunt for food. Plants, lacking this ability, must have some way of procuring food from their immediate surroundings. In highly developed plants, the structures particularly fitted for this purpose are the root, stem and leaf. The root, besides anchoring the plant in the soil, takes in water and minerals. The leaf, being rich in chlorophyll, carries out the process of photosynthesis by uniting the water absorbed by the roots with 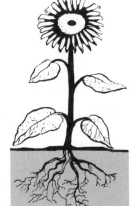 the carbon dioxide from the atmosphere. This process produces simple sugar, an organic food for the plant.

The stem is an intermediate structure which conducts the water from the root to the leaf. It holds the leaf in the best position for it to receive maximum sunlight. The stem also carries the newly manufactured sugar from the leaf to various places in the plant where it can be stored for future use.

Iron Serves Four Distinct Purposes In Plants, Animals and Man

1. Iron produces the chlorophyll (blood) of the plant, principally contained in the green leaves, and the hemoglobin of the red corpuscles in man.

2. Iron enables the plant to take carbon dioxide and nitrogen from the air and to synthesize them into organic matter using chlorophyll and sunlight.

3. Iron assists in the processes of respiration in man and animals. It is the hemoglobin that carries the oxygen to all parts of the body, reaching every cell through the capillaries. Here the carbon of the ingested food, stored in the cells of the tissues, is oxidized and changed into carbonic acid. This in turn is combined with the alkaline elements of the blood and eliminated through the lungs.

4. Iron generates a magnetic blood current and an electromagnetic induction current in the nerve spirals which pass through the walls of the arteries and veins, helping to build and nourish the tissues.

The total amount of iron in the human body is comparatively small. Under normal conditions, it does not exceed 75 grains. Of this quantity, about 50 grains are contained in the blood, with the remainder being distributed throughout the marrow of the bones, in the liver and principally in the spleen. Iron is the most active mineral in the system, and therefore needs to be renewed more frequently than the more stable elements of calcium and potassium in the bones and tissues.

The treatment of diseases should go to the root cause, and most often it is found in severe dehydration from lack of sufficient water, plus an unhealthy lifestyle!

The quantity of blood in a 160 pound normal adult man is about 12 pounds (7.5% of body weight) and contains approximately 50 grains of iron. With every pulse beat, nearly 6 ounces of blood are forced from the heart into our major artery, the aorta. Every 30 seconds, that blood passes from the heart into the lungs. Then the blood travels from the lungs into the arteries and capillaries throughout the body. Consequently, these 50 grains of iron pass through the heart and lungs 120 times per hour, or 2,880 times per day. Within 24 hours under normal conditions, the 50 grains of iron have to perform the same function as 2,880 x 50 grains, or more than 20 pounds! For that reason alone, a daily supply of organic iron in our food is essential to the body.

Vegetables and Fruits are Good Sources of Iron

The best organic iron sources are green leafy vegetables, such as watercress, raw spinach (do not eat cooked spinach since too much oxalic acid is produced by heat), raw parsley, sprouts, raw squash, Swiss chard, dandelion and mustard greens, green cabbage, leeks, nasturtium leaves, sorrel, Bibb lettuce, green lettuce, skins of unwaxed cucumbers, avocado, horseradish, beet greens, artichokes, asparagus, carrots, tomatoes, beets, corn, black radish, pumpkin and corn.

Many fresh organically grown fruits and their juices have a high content of organic iron. Leading the list are blackberries, grapes, cherries, oranges, peaches, raspberries, strawberries, blueberries, gooseberries and pears. Sun-dried natural fruits are high in iron – with apricots being the highest, followed by black figs, prunes, peaches, dates and raisins. Many other foods have a high content of iron: blackstrap and Barbados molasses, raw wheat germ, soy beans, raw and unsalted sesame, pumpkin, sunflower and squash seeds, Brewer's yeast, whole barley, dried beans of all kinds (pinto, kidney, lima, lentils, garbanzos), raw and unsalted nuts, natural brown rice, dried peas, rice bran, wheat bran, rye, whole grain cereals and millet. All these foods will have a higher content of iron if grown organically with no chemical fertilizers and absolutely no poisonous sprays. Let us again impress upon you that your body needs **organic** iron – not the iron that comes from inorganic sources.

Can our bodies get iron from water? You often hear about a certain well or spring containing large amounts of iron. Some water does contain inorganic iron. But your body cannot use this inorganic iron – in fact, this iron is dangerous to your body! It can cause all kinds of stones to form in your vital organs, cement your joints and could turn your blood vessels to stone. Again we caution you: **Stay away from inorganic minerals!**

Every Mineral Matters

The body contains 19 essential mineral elements, all of which must be derived from live food. Calcium, phosphorus and magnesium are vital for the growth and maintenance of bone; potassium, sodium and chlorine give body fluids their composition and stability. Phosphorus, calcium and sulphur are essential constituents of the body cells from which all organs and tissues are composed. Magnesium, iron and phosphorus are vital parts of those enzymes to do with the release of energy from food. Iodine is important to the thyroid gland, which controls growth and the rate at which energy is used. Copper and iron are needed for forming of red blood cells.

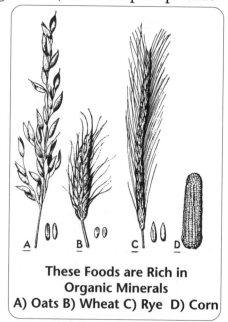

These Foods are Rich in Organic Minerals
A) Oats B) Wheat C) Rye D) Corn

Other minerals like sulphur and cobalt are used in the synthesis of some vitamins by the body. Zinc is an essential part of the insulin molecule. Every mineral contributes a unique factor to vitality, which is the positive proof of good health.

Beets for Longevity

Raw beets and celery have the highest amounts of organic sodium. We eat them almost daily raw in salads and our fresh juices. Once a week we make a beet - veggie combination soup, based on traditional Russian Borscht. We know you'll like this recipe!

BRAGG HEARTY BEET – VEGGIE SOUP
Delicious Hot or Cold!

1½ qts distilled water	1 small onion, minced
2 cups sliced green cabbage	3 cups shredded raw beets
1 cup shredded carrots	1 cup diced celery
2 garlic cloves, minced	2 unpeeled diced potatoes
2 tbsps Virgin Olive Oil	1 tsp Bragg Liquid Aminos
Pinch of Italian Herbs	1 tsp Bragg Organic Apple Cider Vinegar

3 fresh tomatoes (or 1 cup unsalted canned tomatoes)

Mince onion, saute in olive oil for 3 minutes. Add 1½ quarts distilled water and all coarsely shredded veggies. Simmer in covered pot 15 minutes or until veggies are tender. Add tomatoes last 5 minutes. Season with Bragg Liquid Aminos and Organic Raw Apple Cider Vinegar just before serving. We often vary this recipe by adding fresh organic veggies in season, or precooked brown rice, beans, lentils, limas, etc. Serves 4 to 6.

93

As researchers in nutrition and longevity, we have been keenly interested in the long-lived Russians. My father made several expeditions to primitive Russia and found people who lived amazingly long lives – some as old as 140 years! Beets were an important part of their daily diet. They got watercress from fresh mountain streams which they mixed with raw grated beets for a delicious, healthy salad!

Dad found areas where the main sources of water for drinking were rain and snow waters (distilled by Mother Nature) which helps reduce chances of having hardening of the arteries from inorganic minerals and

Soup rejoices the stomach, and prepares it to receive and digest other foods. – Brillat Savarin

To err is human. Admit to your faults, make amends, forgive yourself and learn from your mistakes. It's a wise person who also learns from the mistakes of others.

Health is not quoted in the markets because it is without price.

chemical buildups. Many of these Russians had never tasted common table salt. Their arteries were healthy, flexible, youthful and free from the artery cloggers – inorganic mineral and chemical encrustations!

Salt is a Slow but Sure Killer!

Common table salt (inorganic sodium chloride) is both unnecessary and injurious to the human body. It acts like the inorganic minerals to be found in almost all drinking water except steam-produced distilled water. Table salt can cause encrustations in the arteries, veins and capillaries. It can waterlog body tissues, making them flabby and without skin or muscle tone.

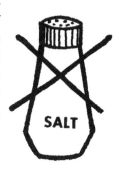

As a general rule, table salt users have a high elevation of blood pessure. According to medical statistics, the Japanese suffer from the highest blood pressure in the world. They are known to be the world's highest salt consumers. And my father's grandfather, who had a massive stroke in front of Dad's eyes at the dinner table, was a heavy user of inorganic salt. He put table salt on everything he ate – including tomatoes, watermelon, cantaloupe, celery and radishes – and he ate many salty foods, including ham, bacon, corned beef, hot dogs, lunch meats, salted popcorn, pretzels and salted nuts.

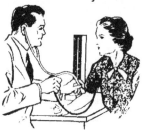

Eating such large amounts of salt and salty foods gave him an unquenchable thirst. My dad would often watch his grandfather consume as much as 2 pitchers of water at each meal! He used table salt, ate salty foods and washed everything down with hard well water that was saturated with inorganic minerals. Is it any wonder that his arteries turned to stone and a stroke killed him?

The unexamined life is not worth living. It is time to re-evaluate your past as a guide to your future. – Socrates

Organic Sodium – Powerful Natural Solvent

Organic sodium is a powerful natural solvent and neutralizer of toxic waste products. In contrast, table salt – an inorganic sodium chloride – not only is unnecessary, but is harmful to the body's chemistry.

In animal and human processes, organic sodium has many important functions. For the transmission of the electric induction current, which is generated in the nerve spirals by iron in the blood, a sodium liquid is necessary (as is shown by the construction of electric batteries). For this purpose, the normal blood serum contains a comparatively large quantity of organic sodium which favors and sustains the generation and conduction of the body's electric currents.

Moreover, organic sodium plays an important part in the formation of saliva, pancreatic juice and bile. The dissolving and reducing properties of sodium can be very distinctly recognized in the emulsification and saponification of fats, especially in the bile. Organic sodium is a fat fighter. It helps to keep the waxy killer, cholesterol, at healthier levels of 150 to 180.

95

Organic sodium is essential for purifying the system of carbonaceous waste products. Let us remind you again that sodium is of value to the body only when obtained in its organic form, as from fruits and vegetables, etc!

Every man is the builder of a temple called his body. We are all sculptors and painters, and our material is our own flesh and blood and bones. Any nobleness begins at once to refine a man's features, any meanness or sensuality to imbrute them. – Henry David Thoreau

The eating of much flesh fills us with a multitude of evil diseases and multitudes of evil desires. – Porphyries, 233 A.D.

It's a little known fact that about 80% of sodium we eat comes not from salt we add at the table or during cooking, but from processed, packaged foods. – Tufts University Nutrition Letter

God makes all things good; man meddles with them and they can become evil. – Rousseau

As previously noted, inorganic salt is indigestible and especially when eaten in large quantities is not easily eliminated from the body. It is therefore deposited in the tissues of the body and an insatiable craving for water develops as the body attempts to wash the salt from its system. Thus the tissues and the vital organs become waterlogged. When this condition reaches the heart, we have what is known as congestive heart failure. The heart cannot function under the combined stress from hardened arteries, added to the flabbiness from waterlogging. Congestive heart failure kills millions!

Misinformation About Killer Salt

Using common table salt is one of the most twisted, widespread habits and injurious to your health! The consumption of salt in the United States now amounts to more than 100 pounds per person each year, and its use is constantly increasing! The salt companies do a thorough brainwashing job, even telling people they need iodized salt to prevent goiter. Sodium chloride, or common table salt, is an inorganic substance which has been the subject of much confusion in the minds of people for many years – particularly in regard to its necessity as an adjunct to our food.

We Constantly Hear These Erroneous Statements About Salt:

- "It is the only substance which we take into our bodies directly from mineral elements."

- "The salt desire is instinctive to humans and animals."

- "Common table salt is one of the most essential of the mineral constituents of the body."

- "In hot weather, when we sweat a great deal, we lose the salt from our bodies. Therefore we should use large amounts of salt and salt tablets to replace it; or else we get sick, weak and suffer from exhaustion."

- "When salt is entirely withheld from an animal, death from salt starvation ensues."

- "Without salt, we would die!"

Salt – a Harmful Preservative. Don't Use It!

All of these assertions, and similar ones, are diametrically opposed to the truth! Why should sodium chloride be an exception among the other inorganic minerals?

Salt has been used in the human diet for thousand of years – but not because the human body needs it! **Salt was the first food preservative discovered by man.** Salt is still used extensively in the preservation of nearly all foods, especially meats and cheeses. It is found in baby foods, canned vegetables, canned fish, prepared cereals, all commercial breads and bakery goods. In fact, it is very hard to find any foods in the supermarkets that have not been contaminated with salt! Even in this modern age of refrigeration and other mechanical marvels, man still craves this primitive use of salt which was used to lengthen the life of his food – and consequently shortens his own!

The salt eating habit is not instinctive. It is acquired, as are the other health-destroying and life-shortening, unhygienic habits, alcohol, smoking, etc. The taste or craving for salt is artificial, because salt paralyzes the 260 taste buds in the mouth. Like any other addiction, salt creates an unnatural craving by deadening certain of the body's warning signals.

97

The advocates of salt point to the animals who often travel miles to the so-called "salt licks." My father studied some of the natural "salt lick" deposits and, on close examination, found little or no sodium!

Cattle, like humans, do not need inorganic sodium. When cattle are fed herbage grown in soils that are poor in mineral elements – especially sodium – such as mountain slopes where rains have carried away the most soluble parts of the soil and deposited them in valleys, they may try to satisfy this deficiency at an artificial (inorganic) "salt-lick."

An animal's taste buds, just like a human's, can be perverted by salt. Often a salt block is put in the pasture so the cattle will lick it, become excessively thirsty and consume large amounts of water. As in humans, the result is waterlogged tissues. Consequently, the cattle ranchers gain profit from waterlogged tissue weight when the cattle are brought to market. Remember, when you eat commercial meat, it may be saturated with inorganic salt, plus other toxins, hormones, etc. Don't make matters worse by adding more table salt to it!

Plenty of fresh fruits, vegetables and salads in your diet will supply your body with all the organic sodium it needs. *For your healthy liquids you will find no purer drink than the unadulterated juice of fresh organic fruits and vegetables and pure distilled water.*

The "Fad" of Drinking Sea Water

From time to time during the past 85 years, some so-called "health experts"have advised drinking sea water to get the minerals which the body requires. They give the argument that billions of tons of top soil are washed into the ocean every year, and that the minerals from this rich soil can be absorbed by the human body to gain more health.

Nothing could be farther from the truth! Yes, the ocean is a vast storehouse of inorganic minerals. But again we must positively state that the human body cannot absorb or utilize any inorganic mineral – whether it comes from a well, spring, river, lake or ocean. Then, too, ocean water has a very high concentration of inorganic sodium chloride (common table salt) which cannot be used by the body chemistry.

Don't drink sea water, no matter what you have been told or read! Sailors and shipwrecked people have tried it many times, and it sent them stark-raving mad to an agonizing death!

Hypertension and fat accumulation in the body are generally the consequences of chronically occurring dehydration. – F. Batmanghelidj, M.D.

According to the Centers for Disease Control, between 900 and 1,000 people a year die and another million people become sick from microbial illnesses from drinking water. Other estimates have put deaths as high as 1,200 and estimated illnesses of more than 7 million, many never reported to doctors.

Sea Salt is Inorganic Sodium (Salt)!

Due to all of the bad publicity about table salt in recent years, many health food stores and manufacturers have begun promoting the use of sea salt. Their rationalization is that this particular form of sodium is healthy and natural since it is coming from the sea. Well, one could make the same argument for common table salt that is taken from the earth via a quarry!

The bottom line is this – no matter where or how on earth it comes from, if salt is not first transformed by plants from inorganic sodium into organic sodium, it cannot be properly absorbed into the body! If you enjoy the taste of salt on your food, then it must come from a plant source.

One option is to sprinkle powdered kelp or dulse over your food. But, perhaps the easiest and healthiest way to get the salty flavor that you like in your foods is to season food with Bragg Liquid Aminos. (See back pages.) Because it's naturally derived from soybeans only, the sodium that it contains is organic, therefore easily absorbed and used by the body. You should avoid using soy or tamari based sauces and seasonings because most of them add inorganic sodium (salt) as well as various artificial flavors, colors, preservatives and other harmful and unnecessary chemicals and additives.

Sea Kelp – Rich Minerals from the Sea

When you eat sea plants such as kelp and seaweed you are following the rules of scientific nutrition. The sea vegetation converts the inorganic minerals of the sea into organic minerals, and it is good to eat most kinds of sea vegetation. We often sprinkle sea kelp on our salads and other foods. It gives the food a tangy flavor and at the same time furnishes the body with natural iodine. In addition to this kelp seasoning of our foods, we take a 5 grain kelp tablet 3 times a week to be assured we get enough organic mineral iodine.

You are what you eat, drink, breathe, think and do! – Patricia Bragg

Overweight and Dropsy

Long before the stage of congestive heart failure is reached, the excessive salt eater suffers from many miseries. The most common of these is overweight and obesity. **Statistics show that 65% of Americans are overweight** – and not all of this is excess fat! Many times overweight is caused by waterlogged tissues. This overweight problem will continue as long as these people use salt on their foods, and especially if they partake freely of salted foods such as canned fish, salted butter, ham, bacon, canned vegetables, cheese, lunch meats, frozen dinners, salted popcorn and nuts. Like hard water, this salt-filled diet damages the arteries, veins and capillaries, as well as the internal organs and tissues of the body.

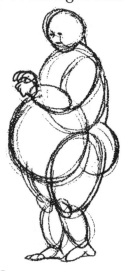

The kidneys are the organs most severely affected by the salt-eating habit. They become weakened and unable to eliminate this large amount of salt, which is then retained in the tissues where, of course, it must be held in solution by water. This condition produces dropsy, which generally occurs in tandem with Bright's disease and cirrhosis. See below for more info about dropsy.

"Dropsy" is a common disease in this country. Observe the ankles of the average person, all too often swollen and puffed-up. This condition is sometimes so severe that their ankles must be bandaged before the afflicted person can stand up. In time, this dropsy becomes chronic and interferes with the circulation to such a degree that leg ulcers or gangrene sets in and an amputation becomes necessary.

OVERWEIGHT, OBESITY, DROPSY AND EDEMA. A person is considered overweight if they are 10 or more pounds above the normal weight for their sex and height; 20% or more above the normal weight is termed obese. Dropsy and edema are caused by an excessive accumulation of fluid in the tissues, leading to swelling. When your body, legs, ankles and feet swell, your heart cannot function correctly.

There are no organs in the body so mercilessly mistreated as the kidneys and liver. Think of the gallons of water saturated with inorganic minerals which these organs try to neutralize! Not only in the water that we drink by itself . . . but water mixed with coffee, tea, alcohol, colas and other soft drinks, plus catsup, mustard and other seasonings with high salt concentrations. Our poor kidneys and liver! What a terrible beating they take! No wonder most people sicken and die long before their time. Man doesn't die: he kills himself by his faulty, unthinking and unhealthy lifestyle!

The World's Greatest Health Secret

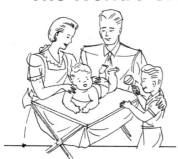

If all babies were to live The Bragg Healthy Lifestyle they would enjoy Long Lives in Painless, Tireless and Ageless Bodies!

101

The "secret" of health lies in **internal cleanliness**! To be 100% healthy, a body must be free from deposits of inorganic minerals that come from drinking city tap water and waters from lakes, rivers, wells and springs. The body is contaminated by inorganic minerals from these sources. Encrustations form that clog and obstruct the body's pipes and impair the vital organs.

The body needs absolutely pure H_2O. Water that comes from raw, organically grown fruits and vegetables is the best life-giving water. It is water that has been charged with solar energy, health-building vitamins, organic minerals and marvelous enzymes! Enzymes can help you build up a natural resistance to any ailment as they help to flush out the accumulated deposits of inorganic minerals and work to dissolve the toxins that are buried deep in your tissues and organs.

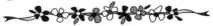

Stomach pains, migraines, allergies, asthma, angina, back and joint pains and even arthritis may all be symptoms of severe dehydration – which can easily be helped by drinking 8 to 10 glasses of pure distilled water every day! Start increasing your water intake today. Be water wise and health safe! – Paul C. Bragg

Fresh Juices are the Magic Cleansers

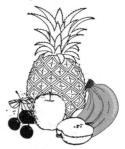

The raw juices of fruits and vegetables are internal cleansers and blood purifiers. These are what we call "the waters of perpetual health and youthfulness." The rays of the sun send billions of atoms into plant life. We can use this solar energy to attain vigorous health, unlimited vitality and physical endurance.

The solar energy from fruits and vegetables can fight the accumulation of inorganic minerals and toxic poisons you have allowed to be deposited in your body. Fruit and vegetable juices are the natural detergents for the human body. Try to get a quart or more of solar energized (freshly-squeezed) fruit and vegetable juices into your body every day.

Go to your Health Store and purchase a juicer and blender. Both of these appliances are important tools in your program of ridding your body of inorganic minerals and toxic wastes. It will probably be the best investment you've ever made! Using a juicer, you can make many varieties of juices. Carrot, celery and raw spinach is a wonderful combination. Carrot, beet and celery make a cocktail rich in organic sodium. Apple and cucumber is a great health cocktail. Green pepper and tomato is a real internal cleanser. Raw spinach and watercress will flood your bloodstream with organic iron. Parsley and carrot is a delicious and healthful combination. Cabbage juice (which Stanford University Medical School discovered helps heal ulcers), onion, garlic, pea-pod, turnip-top, lettuce, kale, dandelion and endive juices are all packed with vital solar energy, vitamins, organic minerals, trace minerals and enzymes.

Fruit juices play an important role in building a clean, healthy bloodstream and body. Organic apple, pineapple, cherry, blackberry, orange, grapefruit, prune, apricot and strawberry juices are the "nectar of the gods".

Healthy, healing dietary fibers are found in fresh vegetables, fresh fruits, salads and whole grains and their products. These health-builders help to normalize blood pressure, weight and cholesterol levels and promote healthy elimination.

Let Natural Food Be Your Medicine

What does food really do in the human body? What relationship does it have with long life and vigorous health – and to disease, misery and physical suffering? How can it be of influence in cleansing the body of inorganic minerals and toxic poisons?

We must have a fundamental, deep understanding of these questions before we can fully appreciate the role diet plays in the maintenance of living processes, the prevention of human diseases, the restoration of health and the prolongation of life.

A balanced diet gives the body nourishment, energy and power. A balanced diet is made up of 60% to 70% raw fruit and vegetables; 20% protein from vegetable sources or, if you insist, animal sources; and equal parts of natural sugars (such as honey), natural starches (such as whole grains or brown rice) and unsaturated fats (such as virgin olive oil, soy, safflower, flaxseed, and hempseed oils). This balanced diet puts your body on the alkaline side and helps to keep the body more internally clean.

103

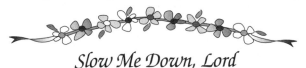

Slow Me Down, Lord

Ease the pounding of my heart by the quieting of my mind.

Steady my hurried pace with a vision of the eternal reach of time.

Give me, amid the confusion of the day, the calmness of the everlasting hills.

Break the tensions of my nerves and muscles with the soothing music of the singing streams that live in my memory. Help me to know the magical, restoring power of sleep.

Teach me the art of taking minute vacations or slowing down to look at a flower, to chat with a friend, to pat a dog, to read a few lines from a good book.

Slow me down, Lord, and inspire me to send my roots deep into the soil of life's enduring values that I may grow toward the stars of my greater destiny.

Re-Educating Your Taste Buds

It will take some willpower to change your habit of eating dead foods to eating live foods. For a while there will be a craving for the unhealthy foods which you have probably eaten all your life. But if you will be positive in your selection of natural foods, the old desire for devitalized foods will soon leave you.

In time, you will find an added pleasure in enjoying the true tastes of the healthy, live foods you eat! You will be able to discern when your 260 taste buds have recovered from salt paralysis and come alive again.

Eliminating Meat is Healthiest

Most uninformed nutritionists call meat the #1 source of protein. Those proteins coming from the vegetable kingdom are referred to as the #2 proteins. This is a sad and terrible mistake. It should be the other way around!

In this day and age, almost all meat is laden with herbicides, fungicides, pesticides and other chemicals that are sprayed on or poured into the feed which these animals consume. They are also pumped full of hormones, antibiotics, growth stimulators and all kinds of drugs to fatten them up and keep them from dying from the extremely unhealthy conditions most of them live in! This is not to mention the admitted fact that many of them are fed the dead, ground up carcasses of other feed lot animals who, for a variety of reasons, didn't make it to the slaughterhouse.

Speaking of the slaughterhouse, what kind of chemical reaction do you suppose would occur in your body if somebody put a choke chain around your neck to keep you in line, shoved you onto a conveyor belt, and made you watch in horror as all of those in line in front of you were beheaded one by one? Well, your body would be pumped so full of adrenaline from all that fear you wouldn't know what hit you! Unused adrenaline is extremely toxic. If you think for a minute that most of the meat that you consume is not packed with this toxic substance, you're sadly mistaken!

Also, consider the fact that cattle, sheep, chickens, etc., are all vegetarians. When you eat them, you are just eating polluted vegetables. Why not skip all the waste and toxins and just eat healthy, organic vegetables?

And what about that myth that you have to eat meat to get your protein? If that were true, where do you suppose farm animals, especially horses, get their protein? They are vegetarians! They get their protein from the grains and grasses that they eat. You are no different. You can get all the proteins you need, and then some, from the organic grains, nuts, seeds, beans, fruits and vegetables that God put on this planet for you to enjoy eating to stay healthy.

Meat is also a major source of uric acid and cholesterol, both harmful to your health. If you are going to include meat in your diet, it should not be eaten more than 3 times a week. In our opinion, fresh fish can be the least toxic of the flesh proteins. But beware of fish from polluted waters. They can be loaded with mercury, lead, cadmium, DDT and many other toxic substances. If you are unable to test the waters from where your fish come, don't risk eating them. And avoid shellfish – shrimp, lobster and crayfish. They are garbage-eating bottom-feeders – the rats and flies of the water kingdom. They eat all of the rotting, decaying scum and refuse off the bottoms of the oceans, lakes and rivers. Next come chicken and turkey – but never eat the skin, which is heavy in cholesterol. Third place goes to lamb and beef.

105

People should not eat pork or pork products of any kind. The pig is the only animal besides man that develops arteriosclerosis or hardening of the arteries. In fact, this animal is so loaded with cholesterol that in cold weather, unprotected pigs and hogs will become solid and stiff, as though frozen solid. Also, this animal is often infected with a dangerous parasite which causes the disease called trichinosis.

We enjoy being vegetarians and not polluting our bodies with unhealthy, meat, fowl and fish proteins. We feel it's safer and healthier getting our proteins from organic vegetables, beans, legumes, nuts, seeds, etc.

% of Calories from Vegetable Proteins

LEGUMES	%
Soybean sprouts	54
Mungbean sprouts	43
Soybean curd (tofu)	43
Soy flour	35
Soybeans	35
Soy sauce	33
Broad beans	32
Lentils	29
Split peas	28
Kidney beans	26
Navy beans	26
Lima beans	26
Garbanzo beans	23

GRAINS	%
Wheat germ	31
Rye	20
Wheat, hard red	17
Wild rice	16
Buckwheat	15
Oatmeal	15
Millet	12
Barley	11
Brown rice	8

FRUITS	%
Lemons	16
Honeydew melon	10
Cantaloupe	9
Strawberry	8
Orange	8
Blackberry	8
Cherry	8
Apricot	8
Grape	8
Watermelon	8
Tangerine	7
Papaya	6
Peach	6
Pear	5
Banana	5
Grapefruit	5
Pineapple	3
Apple	1

VEGETABLES	%
Spinach	49
New Zealand Spinach	47
Watercress	46
Kale	45
Broccoli	45
Brussels Sprouts	44
Turnip Greens	43
Collards	43
Cauliflower	40
Mustard Greens	39
Mushrooms	38
Chinese Cabbage	34
Parsley	34
Lettuce	34
Green Peas	30
Zucchini	28
Green beans	26
Cucumbers	24
Dandelion Greens	24
Green Pepper	22
Artichokes	22
Cabbage	22
Celery	21
Eggplant	21
Tomatoes	18
Onions	16
Beets	15
Pumpkin	12
Potatoes	11
Yams	8
Sweet Potatoes	6

NUTS AND SEEDS	%
Pumpkin seeds	21
Sunflower seeds	17
Walnuts, black	13
Sesame seeds	13
Almonds	12
Cashews	12
Filberts	8

Data obtained from Nutritive Value of American Foods in Common Units, USDA Agriculture Handbook No. 456. Reprinted with author's permission, from *Diet for a New America* by John Robbins (Walpole, NH: Stillpoint Publishing).

106

Avoid These Processed, Refined, Harmful Foods

Once you realize the irreparable harm caused to your body by refined, chemicalized, deficient foods, it is easy to eat correctly. Simply eliminate these "killer" foods from your diet and follow The Bragg Healthy Lifestyle. It provides the basic, essential nourishment your body needs to maintain itself in super energy and health.

• Refined sugar or refined sugar products such as jams, jellies, preserves, marmalades, yogurts, ice cream, sherbets, Jello, cake, candy, cookies, chewing gum, soft drinks, pies, pastries, tapioca puddings and all sugared fruit juices and fruits canned in sugar syrup. (Health stores have healthy, delicious replacements, so seek, buy and enjoy!)

• White flour products such as white bread, wheat-white bread, enriched flours, rye bread that has white flour in it, dumplings, biscuits, buns, gravy, pasta, pancakes, waffles, soda crackers, pizza, ravioli, pies, pastries, cakes, cookies, prepared and commercial puddings and ready-mix bakery products. (Health Stores have a huge variety of 100% whole grain products – delicious breads, crackers, pastas, pizzas, pastries, etc.)

• Salted foods, such as corn and potato chips, crackers and nuts.

• White rice and pearled barley.   • Fried and greasy foods.

• Commercial, highly processed dry cereals made from corn, oats, etc.

• Food that contains palm and cottonseed oil. Products labeled vegetable oil . . . find out what kind before you use them.

107

• Peanuts and peanut butter that contains hydrogenated, hardened oils and any mold that causes allergies.

• Margarine – full of dangerous, unnatural, trans-fatty acids.

• Saturated fats and hydrogenated oils – enemies that clog the bloodstream.

• Coffee, decaffeinated coffee, China black tea and all alcoholic beverages. Also all caffeinated and sugared cola and soft drinks.

• Fresh pork and pork products.   • Fried, fatty and greasy meats.

• Smoked meats, such as ham, bacon, sausage and smoked fish.

• Luncheon meats, hot dogs, salami, bologna, corned beef, pastrami and packaged meats containing dangerous sodium nitrate or nitrite.

• Dried fruits containing sulphur dioxide – a preservative.

• Do not eat chickens or turkeys that have been injected with stilbestrol or fed with poultry feed that contains any drugs.

• Canned soups - read labels for sugar, starch, flour and preservatives.

• Food that contains benzoate of soda, salt, sugar, cream of tartar . . . and any other additives, drugs or preservatives.

• Day-old cooked vegetables, potatoes and pre-mixed, wilted salads.

• Pasteurized, filtered vinegars, distilled white, malt and synthetic vinegars – these are the dead vinegars! (We use only organic, raw, unfiltered apple cider vinegar with the "mother" as used in olden times.)

BENEFITS FROM THE JOYS OF FASTING

Fasting is easier than any diet. • Fasting is the quickest way to lose weight.
Fasting is adaptable to a busy life. • Fasting gives the body a physiological rest.
Fasting is used successfully in the treatment of many physical illnesses.
Fasting can yield weight losses of up to 10 pounds or more in the first week.
Fasting lowers & normalizes cholesterol and blood pressure levels.
Fasting is a calming experience, often relieving tension and insomnia.
Fasting improves dietary habits. • Fasting increases eating pleasure.
Fasting frequently induces feelings of euphoria, a natural *high.*
Fasting is a rejuvenator, slowing the ageing process.
Fasting is an energizer, not a debilitator. • Fasting aids the elimination process.
Fasting often results in a more vigorous sex life.
Fasting can eliminate or modify smoking, drug and drinking addictions.
Fasting is a regulator, educating the body to consume food only as needed.
Fasting saves time spent marketing, preparing and eating.
Fasting rids the body of toxins, giving it an "internal shower" & cleansing.
Fasting does not deprive the body of essential nutrients.
Fasting can be used to uncover the sources of food allergies.
Fasting is used effectively in schizophrenia treatment & other mental illnesses.
Fasting under proper supervision can be tolerated easily up to 4 weeks.
Fasting does not accumulate appetite; hunger "pangs" disappear in 1-2 days.
Fasting is routine for the animal kingdom.
Fasting has been a commonplace experience since man's existence.
Fasting is a rite in all religions; the Bible alone has 74 references to it.
Fasting under proper conditions is absolutely safe.
Fasting is not starving, it's nature's cure that God has given us. – Patricia Bragg
        – Allan Cott, M.D., *Fasting As A Way Of Life*

108

Spiritual Bible Reasons Why We Should Fast
For a Healthier, Happier, Longer Walk With Our Creator

3 John 2	Deut. 11:7-15,21	Luke 9:11	Matthew 9: 9-15
Gen. 6:3	Gal. 5:13-26	Mark 2:16-20	Neh. 9:1, 20-24
I Cor. 7:5	Isaiah 58	Matthew 4:1-4	Psalms 35:13
II Cor. 6	James 5:10-20	Matthew 6:6-18	Romans 16:16-20
Deut. 8:3	John 15	Matthew 7	Zachariah 8:1

Dear HEALTH FRIEND,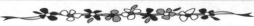

This gentle reminder explains the great benefits from *The Miracle of Fasting* that you will enjoy when starting on your weekly, 24 hour, Bragg Fasting Program for Super Health! It's a precious time of body-mind-soul cleansing and renewal.

On fast days I drink 7 to 10 glasses of distilled water, some with ACV and you also may have some herbal teas and if needed diluted fresh juices (dilute with 3 distilled water). Every day, even some fast days, you may add 1 tbsp. of this mixture (2 oat bran and 2 psyllium husk powder) to liquids twice a day. It's an extra cleanser and helps normalize weight, cholesterol and blood pressure and helps promote healthy elimination. Fasting is the oldest, most effective healing method known to man. Fasting offers great, miraculous blessings from Mother Nature and our Creator. It begins the self-cleansing of the inner-body workings so we can promote our own self-healing.

My father and I wrote the book *The Miracle of Fasting* to share with you the health miracles it can perform in your daily life. It's all so easy to do and it's an important part of The Bragg Healthy Lifestyle.

                             With Love, *Patricia*

Paul Bragg's work on fasting and water is one of the great contributions to the Healing Wisdom and the Natural Health Movement in the world today.
– Gabriel Cousens, M.D., Author, Conscious Eating and Spiritual Nutrition

Fasting Cleanses, Renews and Rejuvenates

There is a natural self-cleansing and healing system for maintaining a healthy body and our "river of life" – our bloodstream. It's essential that we keep our entire bodily machine in perfect health from head to toes and in good working order to maintain life!

Fasting is the best detoxifying method. It's also the most effective and safest way to increase elimination of waste buildups and enhance the body's miraculous self-healing and self-repairing process that keeps you healthy.

If you prepare for a fast by eating a cleansing diet for 1 to 2 days, this can greatly facilitate the cleansing process. Fresh variety salads, fresh vegetables and fruits and their juices, as well as green drinks (alfalfa, barley, chlorophyll, chlorella, spirulina, wheatgrass, etc.) stimulate waste elimination. Live, fresh foods and juices can literally pick up dead matter from your body and carry it away. After this pre-cleansing diet you can start your liquid fast.

Daily, even on most days during our fasts, we take 3,000 mg. of mixed vitamin C powder (C concentrate, acerola, rosehips and bioflavonoids) in liquids. This is a potent antioxidant and it flushes out deadly free radicals. It also promotes collagen production for new healthy tissues. Vitamin C is especially important if you are detoxifying from prescription drugs or alcohol overload.

109

Either a moderate and well-planned distilled water fast (our favorite) or, if easier for you, a diluted fresh juice fast (⅓ distilled water) can cleanse your body of excess mucus, old fecal matter, trapped cellular and non-food wastes. These fasts help remove inorganic mineral deposits and sludge from your pipes and joints. Fasting works by self-digestion. During a fast, your body will intuitively decompose and burn only the substances and tissues that are damaged, diseased or unneeded, such as abscesses, tumors, excess fat deposits, excess water and congestive wastes.

U.S. Constitution Inspired by Fasting and Prayer in 1787

In 1787, representatives of the 13 states gathered in Philadelphia to create the Constitution. Dissension and disputes among the delegates nearly ended the convention. It was then that Benjamin Franklin, the great statesman, intervened with the most extraordinary speech anyone had delivered in the entire three months the delegates had been meeting. He said, "The longer I live, the more I am convinced that God governs in the affairs of man. I therefore move we begin each session in prayer, asking the assistance of heaven and its blessing on our deliberations." They immediately declared three days of prayer and fasting to seek God's help in breaking the deadlock. At the end of that time all resentments and wrangling were gone and at last the delegates began working together to write a constitution for the United States of America.

Even a relatively short fast (1 to 3 days) will accelerate elimination from your liver, kidneys, lungs, bloodstream and skin. Sometimes you will experience dramatic changes, which we call cleansing and healing crises, as accumulated wastes are expelled. With your first fasts you may temporarily have headaches, fatigue, body odor, bad breath, coated tongue, mouth sores and even diarrhea as your body is cleaning house. Please be patient and loving with your body – your miracle home!

After a fast, your body will begin to self-cleanse and healthfully rebalance! When you follow The Bragg Healthy Lifestyle, your weekly 24-hour fast removes toxins on a regular basis so they don't accumulate! Your energy levels will soon begin to rise – physically, psychologically and mentally. Your creativity will begin to expand. You will feel like a "different person" – which you are – you are being cleansed, purified and reborn! It's an exciting and wonderful miracle that is happening!

Master Key to Internal Purification

If you do a complete water fast for 24 hours each week, soon you will be able to add more fresh fruit and vegetables to your diet. After fasting 3 or more days, you can include more foods in a high rate of vibration.

I faithfully fast for 24 hours every Monday and the first three days of each month. Wait until you experience this! You will greatly benefit from the inner cleansing and will love the pure, clean, healthy feeling you receive!

Fasting Brings Remarkable Results

Professor A.E. Crews of Edinburgh University, who studied both worms and animals, stated: *"Given appropriate and essential conditions of the environment, including proper care of the body . . . Eternal Youth, in fact, can be a reality in living forms! It's found to be possible, by repeated processes of fasting, to keep a worm alive twenty times longer than it would have lived in the regular way. This has also been proven with animals."* Life-extending results have been proven again in a recently published earthworm study. Something to think about, indeed, that proves the merits of fasting for humans!

Food and Product Summary

Today, many of our foods are highly processed or refined, which robs them of essential nutrients, vitamins, minerals and enzymes. Many also contain harmful and dangerous chemicals. The research findings and experience of top nutritionists, physicians and dentists have led to the discovery that devitalized foods are a major cause of poor health, illness, cancer and premature death. The enormous increase in the last 70 years of degenerative diseases such as heart disease, arthritis and dental decay substantiate this belief. Scientific research has shown that most of these afflictions can be prevented and that others, once established, may be arrested or even reversed through nutritional methods.

Enjoy Super Health with Natural Foods

1. **RAW FOODS:** Use fresh fruits and raw vegetables (organically grown is always best). Have nutritious variety garden salads with sprouts and raw nuts and seeds.

2. **VEGETABLE and ANIMAL PROTEINS:**
   a. Legumes, brown rice, soy and beans – *our favorites.*
   b. Nuts and seeds, raw and unsalted.
   c. Animal protein (if you must) – hormone free meats, liver, kidney, brain, heart, poultry, seafood. Please eat these proteins sparingly or best to enjoy the healthier vegetarian diet. You can bake, roast, wok or broil your animal proteins. Eat no more than 3 times weekly.
   d. Dairy products – eggs (fertile), unprocessed hard cheese, goat's cheese and certified raw milk. (Personally we do not use milk and only occasionally unsalted butter. Try soy, nut and rice milks – our favorite.

3. **FRUITS and VEGETABLES:** Organically grown is always best – grown without the use of poisonous sprays and toxic chemical fertilizers whenever possible; ask your market to stock organic produce. Steam, bake, saute or wok veggies for as short a time as possible to retain the best nutritional content and flavor. Also enjoy fresh juices.

4. **100% WHOLE GRAIN CEREALS, BREADS and FLOURS:** They contain important B-complex vitamins, vitamin E, minerals and the important unsaturated fatty acids.

5. **COLD or EXPELLER-PRESSED VEGETABLE OILS:** Virgin olive oil, sunflower, flax and sesame oils are excellent sources of the healthy, essential, unsaturated fatty acids; but it's still wise to use all oils sparingly.

These freshly squeezed organic vegetable and fruit juices are important to The Bragg Healthy Lifestyle. It's not wise to drink beverages with your main meals, as it dilutes the digestive juices. But it's great during the day to have a glass of freshly squeezed orange, grapefruit, vegetable juice, Bragg Vinegar Drink, herb tea or try a hot cup of Bragg Liquid Aminos Broth (½ to 1 tsp Bragg Liquid Aminos in cup of hot distilled water) – these are all ideal pick-me-up beverages.

Bragg Apple Cider Vinegar Cocktail – Mix 1-2 tsp. equally of Bragg Organic ACV and raw honey (optional) in glass of distilled water. Take 1 glass upon arising, 1 an hour before lunch and 1 an hour before dinner.

Delicious Hot Cider Drink – Add a few cinnamon sticks and cloves to hot distilled water and let steep for 20 mins. Before drinking add 2 tsps of Bragg Raw Organic Apple Cider Vinegar and raw honey equally.

Bragg Favorite Juice Cocktail – This drink consists of all raw vegetables (please remember organic is best) which we prepare in our vegetable juicer: carrots, celery, beets, cabbage, watercress and parsley. The great purifier, garlic we enjoy but it's optional.

Bragg Favorite Healthy "Pep" Drink – After our morning stretch and exercises we often enjoy this instead of fruit. It's also delicious and powerfully nutritious as a meal anytime: lunch, dinner or take along in a thermos to work, school, the gym, or to the park or hiking, etc.

Bragg Healthy Pep Drink

Prepare the following in blender, add 1 ice cube if desired colder:
Choice of: freshly squeezed orange juice, grapefruit or tangelo; carrot and greens juice; unsweetened pineapple juice; or 1 ½ cups distilled water with:

½ tsp raw wheat germ	*¼ tsp vitamin C powder*
⅓ tsp flaxseed oil, optional	*¼ tsp nutritional yeast flakes*
¼ tsp green powder (barley, etc.)	*1 to 2 bananas, ripe*
½ tsp raw oat bran	*1 tsp raw honey, optional*
½ tsp psyllium husk powder	*1 tsp soy protein powder*
½ tsp lecithin granules	*1 tsp raw sunflower seeds*

Optional: 4 apricots (sun dried, unsulphured). Soak in jar overnight in distilled water or unsweetened pineapple juice. We soak enough to last for several days. Keep refrigerated. In summer, you can add fresh fruit in season: peaches, strawberries, berries, apricots, etc. instead of the banana. In winter, add apples, oranges, pears or persimmons or try sugar-free, frozen organic fruits. Serves 1 to 2.

Patricia's Delicious Health Popcorn

Use freshly popped popcorn (I prefer air popped). If desired, use olive, soy, or safflower oil or melted salt-free butter. Pour the oil over popcorn and then add several sprays of Bragg Liquid Aminos. Sprinkle with nutritional yeast flakes or grated parmesan cheese. For variety, add pinch of Italian or French herbs, cayenne pepper, mustard powder or fresh crushed garlic to the oil mixture. Delicious served instead of breads!

Super Powered Lentil & Brown Rice Casserole

14 oz pkg lentils, uncooked
4 carrots, chopped
3 celery stalks, chopped
2 onions, chopped
3 quarts distilled water

4 garlic cloves, chopped
1 cup brown rice, uncooked
1 tsp Bragg Liquid Aminos
¼ tsp Italian herbs (oregano, basil, etc.)
2 tsp olive oil (virgin - cold-pressed is best)

Wash & drain lentils and rice. Place grains in large stainless steel pot. Add water. Bring to boil, reduce heat & simmer for 30 minutes. Add vegetables & seasonings & cook on low heat until done. Just before serving, you may add fresh or canned tomatoes. For a delicious garnish add parsley & nutritional yeast large flakes. Add more water in cooking the grains to make this recipe a delicious soup or stew. Serves 4 to 6.

Bragg Raw Vegetable Garden Salad

2 stalks celery, chopped
1 bell pepper & seeds, diced
½ cucumber, chopped
1 carrot, grated
1 raw beet, grated
1 cup green cabbage, sliced

½ cup red cabbage, chopped
½ cup alfalfa or sunflower sprouts
2 spring onions & tops, chopped
1 turnip, grated
1 avocado (ripe)
3 tomatoes, medium size

For variety add raw zucchini, sugar peas, mushrooms, broccoli, cauliflower. Dice avocado & tomato and serve on side as a dressing. Chop, slice or grate vegetables fine to medium for variety in size. Mix vegetables thoroughly & serve on a bed of lettuce, spinach, watercress or chopped cabbage. Serve choice of fresh squeezed lemon, orange or dressing separately. Chill salad plates before serving. Always eat your salad first before serving hot dishes. Serves 3 to 5.

Bragg Vinaigrette Health Dressing

½ cup Bragg Apple Cider Vinegar   *⅓ tsp Bragg Liquid Aminos*
2 tsps raw honey   *1 to 2 cloves garlic, minced*
⅓ cup virgin olive oil, or blend with safflower, soy or sesame
1 Tbsp fresh herbs, minced or pinch Italian or French dry herbs

Blend ingredients in blender or jar. Refrigerate in covered jar.
For delicious herbal vinegar: in quart jar add ⅓ cup tightly packed, crushed fresh sweet basil, tarragon, dill, oregano, or any fresh herbs desired, combined or singly. (If *dried* herbs, use 1 to 2 tsp. herbs.) Now cover to top with Bragg Organic Raw Apple Cider Vinegar and store 2 weeks in warm place, strain and refrigerate.

Honey–Celery Seed Vinaigrette

¼ tsp dry mustard
¼ tsp Bragg Liquid Aminos
¼ tsp paprika
3 Tbsp raw honey

1 cup Bragg Apple Cider Vinegar
½ cup virgin olive oil
1 medium onion, minced
⅓ tsp celery seed

Blend ingredients in blender or jar. Refrigerate in covered jar.

Healthy, organic foods have a wonderful abundance of potential life energy.

Healthy Foods Naturally Rich
In Important Vitamin E for Your Health

This is a list of foods that contain the following notable amounts of precious, healthy Vitamin E. This list was compiled from *Bridges Food and Beverage Analyses.*

Food	Quantity	Vitamin E IU's
Apples	1 medium	0.74
Bananas	1 medium	0.40
Barley	½ cup	4.20
Beans, Navy	½ cup	3.60
Butter (salt-free)	6 tablespoons	2.40
Carrots	1 cup	0.45
Celery, Green	½ cup	2.60
Corn, Dried for Popcorn	1 cup	20.00
Cornmeal, Yellow	½ cup	1.70
Corn Oil	6 tablespoons	87.00
Eggs, Fertile	2	2.00
Endive, Escarole	½ cup	2.00
Flour, Whole Grain	1 cup	54.00
Grapefruit	½	0.52
Kale	½ cup	8.00
Lettuce	6 leaves	0.50
Oatmeal	½ cup	2.00
Olive Oil (virgin)	½ cup	5.00
Onions, Raw	2 medium	0.26
Oranges	1 small	0.24
Parsley	½ cup	5.50
Peas, Green	1 cup	4.00
Potatoes, White	1 medium	0.06
Potatoes, Sweet	1 small	4.00
Rice, Brown	1 cup cooked	2.40
Rye	½ cup	3.00
Soybean Oil	6 tablespoons	140.00
Sunflower Seeds, Raw	½ cup	31.00
Wheatgerm Oil	6 tablespoons	50 – 420.00

114

There are 54 Healthy Salad Recipes & 23 Delicious Dressing Recipes in the 448 page Bragg *Gourmet Recipes Book.* *See back pages for booklist.*

A recent study of nurses whose daily Vitamin E intake was 100 mgs and more had a 36% lower risk of heart attack and 23% lower risk of stroke.

Chapter 6

The Water We Need for Health

Drink Only Distilled Water

Other than the fruit and vegetable juices, my father and I drink no other liquid except steam-produced distilled water. Today, in this polluted and poisoned world, distilled water is the purest water on the face of the earth. It contains no solid matter of any kind. It is made solely of two elements, hydrogen and oxygen. There are no minerals in it, organic or inorganic. It can be used as drinking water and cooking water and also can be used in electric steam irons, batteries, etc.

When distilled water enters the body, it leaves no residue of any kind. It's free of salt and sodium. It's also the most perfect water to promote healthy functioning of those great "sieves," the kidneys. It's the perfect liquid for the blood. It's the ideal liquid for efficient functioning of the lungs, stomach, liver and all your organs.

Why? Because it's free of all inorganic minerals! It's so pure that all liquid drug prescriptions are formulated with distilled water.

Let no person tell you that distilled water is dead water! Of course, fish will not live in distilled water. Fish require vegetable growth in water and vegetable growth needs inorganic minerals to live.

What About Rain Water?

Rain water once was the ideal distilled water. Today, most air has some pollution that poisons and contaminates this natural water. It's a theory of ours that the amazing people mentioned in the Bible who lived to fantastic ages drank only rain water. Rain water is distilled water from the clouds.

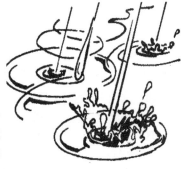

However, we now live in the age of pollution when even the rains from above are contaminated! Such toxins as Strontium 90 from atomic bombs and the exhaust from airplanes and automobiles turn rain water into a deadly poison. Vicious toxins are sent into the air from our industrial factories – sulfur dioxides, lead, carbon monoxide and hundreds of pollutants.

So, in our present civilization, drinking rain water is out of the question! To live in this poisoned world, to survive and to save ourselves from another kind of destruction (the complete solidification of the body, brain structures, etc.), please drink only distilled water.

We do not want our brain, arteries and other blood vesels to turn into stone! You see this condition every day in prematurely old people suffering from deep senility, Alzheimer's, etc. Often you hear the word "fossil" used to describe the prehistoric remnants of animals who lived on earth ages ago. When you drink a glass of ordinary tap water, the process of fossilization has already begun. When a person dies of hardening of the arteries, he has reached the ultimate end.

So many times we've heard someone say something such as, "That old fossil John Smith died last night from hardening of the arteries." Although the remark was crude, it was truthful! If we escape the other deadly degenerative and infectious diseases in this life, we are always haunted by that great killer of mankind, "hardening of the arteries."

How to Fight Hardening of the Arteries

Be determined that you are going to drink only pure distilled water. If you cannot get it delivered from a water company, try the health or grocery store. Also, drug stores carry distilled water for people who have heart trouble or strokes. Don't wait until these happen to you!

If you cannot find distilled water for sale anywhere, then purchase a small still and distill your own water. You may say that is a lot of trouble – but it's not nearly as much trouble as when your arteries start to harden and your body is slowly starved for want of oxygen!

Remember, the bloodstream carries oxygen to all parts of the body. And if the arteries become encrusted with inorganic minerals, you are in for grave problems. Oxygen starvation causes a host of serious ailments.

Stages of Artery Hardening

This drawing shows the 3 stages of the hardening of blood vessels in the brain. As the flow of blood becomes slower, clots may form and completely close a vessel.

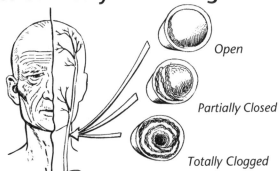

Open

Partially Closed

Totally Clogged

We Drink Juices During Our World Health Crusades

At times we are unable to find distilled water during our many Bragg Health Crusades which carry us around the world. But when it is not available – or if we are in doubt about the water supply – for short perods we let fresh raw vegetables, fruits and their juices supply us with their naturally pure water. We always have a small hand citrus juicer with us for our fresh orange or grapefruit juice. Fresh is always best!

The Great Watermelon Flush

There is nothing like a watermelon flush to dissolve and eliminate inorganic minerals from your body.

As a youth, my father had a history of drinking exceptionally hard water, loaded with inorganic minerals. The contaminants in that hard water encrusted the pipes of his body, and when he learned the truth of the great damage it could do to his system, he started to experiment with fruits and vegetables to find out which one had the greatest encrustation-dissolving power. It was a long search, but at last he found it! Watermelon and its juice does the cleansing miracle.

Man is as old as his arteries. – Virchow

Several times a year we both go on a watermelon flush. We eat nothing for 5 to 7 days but watermelon and watermelon juice. Every morning we take a sample of the very first urine we void. We seal it tightly, date it and put it on a shelf for 6 months to a year. As it breaks down, the inorganic minerals, which are heavier, settle on the bottom of the bottle. Being a biochemist, my father has thoroughly analyzed these substances and found calcium carbonate, magnesium carbonate and many other inorganic minerals, chemicals and toxins.

That is why we go on a watermelon flush several times a year and often will make it our lunch meal. It's best not to mix melons with other foods. We also eat watermelon all during its season. Many times we have paid high prices for watermelon to be shipped from warm climates during the winter months, but we just consider that good health insurance. On an average day in the hot summertime, we will drink as much as 1 to 2 quarts of watermelon juice.

The result is that Dad has the blood pressure of a man of 25 – it is 120 over 80 and his pulse is around 60. We both have our heart and arteries examined by a heart specialist every year. So far there is not the slightest sign of any hardening of our arteries. We can jog, run, swim and ride our bikes for miles. We both have supple, flexible arteries and blood vessels. There are no big, bulging veins on our foreheads, such as we've seen on people a third of our calendar years! We can stand on our heads for 15 minutes at a time with absolutely no dizziness or other reaction. We also have perfect hearing. We live as we teach and this healthy lifestyle fights the body's worst enemy – hardening of the arteries. We both expect to live a long, happy, active, healthy life!

There are no more important ingredients of a properly constituted diet than organic fruits and vegetables, for they contain vitamins and minerals of every class, recognized and unrecognized. – Sir Robert McCarrison

One solution to America's soaring health costs is pure distilled water.

The body and the mind are so closely connected that not even a single word or thought can come into existence without being reflected in the personality and health of the individual. – John Prentiss

Paul C. Bragg's Prediction

Mine is only a small voice in the wilderness concerning this matter of drinking only distilled water, but I sincerely wish to save humanity from the dangers of water filled with chemicals and inorganic minerals.

I have lived a long life. During this time I have seen my relatives and my personal friends, as well as some very fine animals, die of fossilization.

I believe I am a hundred years ahead of my time in my theories on the dangers of inorganic water. Someday humanity will recognize the dangers in ordinary water and all the water used in homes, schools, hospitals, etc. will be steam distilled! It will be the greatest health advancement this "modern" world has ever known!

No matter how much a person controls his eating habits . . . no matter how much juice of organic fruits and vegetables he drinks, no matter if he lives on a raw food, vegetarian or so-called modern scientific diet . . . as long as he continues to drink spring, well, river, lake or fluoridated and chlorinated water he is going to fossilize himself! In the past 85 years I have met all the greats in the field of nutrition, natural healing, etc., but they all drank the deadly, inorganically mineralized water – and only a very few of them have attained an extra long, healthy life.

The same is true of the great athletes of the past 85 years. They had their day in the sun, drank the deadly inorganic mineral water and died at about the same age as non-athletic people.

I was personally acquainted with Bill Tilden, the greatest tennis player of all time. In his prime, no man in the world could defeat him. But he would not listen to my lone, small voice when I told him of the viciousness and deadliness of inorganic drinking water. He said that everybody else was drinking ordinary water, so he saw no reason why he should stop. All his athletic

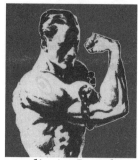

strength and prowess didn't save him from having a massive coronary. He died before he was 60! The autopsy showed that his arteries were like stone.

Sandow, the greatest strong man of all times, was a friend of mine. When I would visit him in his studio in London, England, he would flex his muscles and tell me how powerful he was. But he drank London tap water and at 58 he also had a massive coronary. His great strength and bulging muscles could not save his life. Man is as old as his arteries! There is absolutely no way to circumvent this powerful truth.

For example: during the Korean war approximately 300 young American soldiers were killed within a short period. Autopsies were performed upon all of them. And what do you think was revealed? That these young men all showed signs of hardening of the arteries! This scientific study is on record. These were young men under 23, in the so-called prime of life, suffering from degeneration (fossilizing) of the body's arteries.

Life Expectancy – Life Span

We are told that a male child born today has a life expectancy of 72 years, and a female about 78. What is the actual life span of the average American? A male child about 65 years, and a female child about 69 years.

So we can see that when a male reaches 33 years he has lived about half of his lifetime, and when a female reaches 34 years she has lived about half of her lifetime. The sad but true fact is that some people, if not most, never even reach their expected life span.

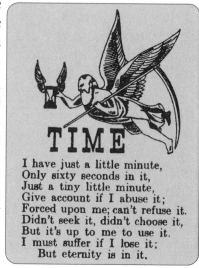

TIME

I have just a little minute,
Only sixty seconds in it,
Just a tiny little minute,
Give account if I abuse it;
Forced upon me; can't refuse it.
Didn't seek it, didn't choose it,
But it's up to me to use it.
I must suffer if I lose it;
But eternity is in it.

The U.S. and other western countries are experiencing an epidemic of heart disease and cancer. Consider this startling fact: chances are better than 2 to 1 that, directly or indirectly, the average American adult will die of some form of heart disease or cancer.

You as an individual can reverse this shocking statistic by avoiding ordinary water that is laced with inorganic minerals and toxins, stop using salt, reducing saturated fatty foods, exercising regularly, drinking only distilled water and eating a balanced, healthy diet.

Exercise is Vital for Health and Longevity

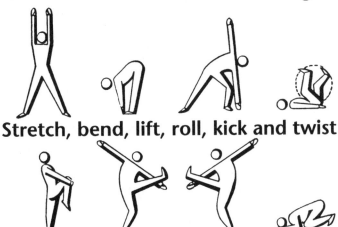

Stretch, bend, lift, roll, kick and twist

121

For youthful arteries, exercise is essential! If you wish to live a long, healthy life it is necessary to build up your cardiovascular endurance and to follow a program designed to keep your arteries soft and agile.

The first step is to get more oxygen into the body which will help dissolve the encrustations that have formed in the arteries. Any physical activity that injects more oxygen is going to help extend your life! Get out and jog, swim, ride a bike or take a brisk 2 to 3 mile healthy walk.

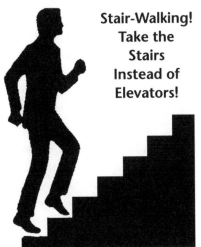

Stair-Walking! Take the Stairs Instead of Elevators!

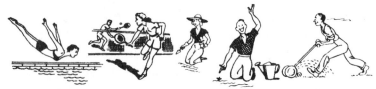

Keep Young Biologically with Exercise and Good Nutrition

Why grow old? Why not grow biologically younger as you live longer? Don't let parts of your wonderful body become fossilized by drinking inorganic mineral water! Aim for healthy perfection and protect your body!

Be the Health Captain of Your Life!

Please don't drink chemicalized or inorganically mineralized waters. Don't eat foods that your judgment tells you should not be eaten! Be stronger than your physical cravings! Do not give in to any temptation and you will soon find that the inclination will vanish. The really healthy man is always able to rule his flesh and desires! The greatest triumph is the victory over self!

Don't be afraid of being called a "crank" or "faddist" because you wish to live abundantly through regulation of your drinking and eating habits. There probably has never been a change that brought abundant blessings to humanity which was not ridiculed at first!

Follow The Bragg Healthy Lifestyle!
Here are some good reasons why you should:

- It reflects the ironclad laws of Mother Nature.
- Your common sense, which tells you that you are doing the right thing.
- You are working to make your health better and your life longer.
- Your resolve to prevent illness so that you may enjoy a healthy life to its fullest.
- By making an art of your life, you will remain youthful at any calendar age.
- You will retain your faculties and be hale, hearty, active and useful far beyond the ordinary length of years.
- You will possess superior mental and physical powers.

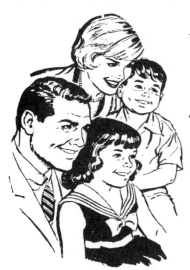

Life's Greatest Treasure is Radiant Health

"There is no substitute for Health!
Those who possess it
are richer than kings."
– Paul C. Bragg

Comfort, Security and Happiness for You

Can you think of any greater comfort than the confidence that you will not be the victim of inorganic minerals, toxic poisons and harmful chemicals? That you will be able to keep these killers out of your body?

Would it not be a wonderful comfort to you to have this great anxiety removed from your life? How glorious to feel the positive conviction that you can live a long vibrant, active, healthy life! Think of how blessed you'll be once you can teach your children, your relatives and friends how to live in comfort, secure against all preventable human miseries and untimely death!

Surely the removal of this incredible anxiety from our minds seems "too good to be true." Yet this delightful state of affairs is not only possible, but is easily attainable by anyone willing to apply the healthy lifestyle principles given in this book.

We can tell you from our hearts with the strongest conviction that we firmly believe that all manner of illness and misery is wholly of our own making. Prevent ill health by avoiding all chemicalized and inorganic mineral water; by keeping away from table salt; by practicing healthy dietary habits; by not smoking and by having a consistent program of exercise.

Drinking 8 glasses daily of pure distilled water helps cleanse, purify, renew and recharge our human batteries, to insure a longer, healthier, happier life! – Paul C. Bragg

How Safe is Chlorinated Water?

An estimated 75% of drinking water in the U.S. is chlorinated. While chlorination has helped to reduce the incidence of infectious diseases, known carcinogens such as chloroform and other trihalomethanes are formed when chlorine reacts with organic compounds in the water. These chlorines accumulate in fatty tissue such as breast tissues and can be found in body fat, blood, mothers' milk and semen. Studies have implicated chlorinated drinking water with colorectal and bladder cancers. Highly chlorinated water resulted in a noticeable shift in the transformation of cholesterol from beneficial HDL to harmful LDL.

Recently, the American Journal of Public Health published the results of a study of cancer risk over an 8 year period in 28,237 postmenopausal women. Those who drank water from municipal surface water sources consumed higher levels of chloroform than those who drank municipal ground water sources. The higher intake of chloroform was associated with an increased risk of colon cancer, and of all cancers combined.

"The worldwide pollution of lakes, streams, rivers and oceans and the chlorination of swimming pool water has led to an increase in deadly melanoma."

– Reports Franz Rampen in *Epidemiology*

Even chlorination does not provide full protection against the deadliest organisms in public water supplies. Cryptosporidium, a toxic parasitic protozoan, is chlorine resistant and inadequately removed by sand filters.

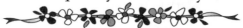

The power of pure water is the vital chemistry of life!

The laws of health are inexorable; we see people going down and out in their prime of life because no attention is paid to them! – Paul C. Bragg

Water, the solvent of the body, regulates all body functions, including the eliminations of toxins and body waste.

Dehydration causes stress, and stress will cause further dehydration.
– F. Batmanghelidj, M.D. author of
Your Body's Many Cries for Water; You Are Not Sick, You Are Thirsty!

20 FACTS ABOUT DISTILLED WATER

You should know that Distilled Water . . .

- is water that has been turned into vapor so that its impurities are left behind. Upon condensing, it becomes pure water.
- is the only type of water which meets the definition of water; hydrogen + oxygen.
- is a perfectly natural water.
- is also odorless, colorless and tasteless.
- is free of virtually all inorganic minerals including salt.
- is the only natural solvent that can be taken into the body without damage to the tissues.
- acts as a solvent in the body by dissolving nutrients so they can be assimilated and taken into every cell.
- dissolves the cell wastes so the toxins can be removed.
- dissolves inorganic mineral substances lodged in the tissues of the body so that such substances can be eliminated in the process of purifying the body.
- does not leach out organic body minerals but does collect and remove the toxic inorganic minerals which have been rejected by the cells of the body and are therefore nothing more than harmful debris obstructing the normal functions of the body.

125

- is indeed the most ideal and beneficial water for all humans and also for animals.
- leaves no residue of any kind when it enters the body.
- is the most perfect water for the healthy functioning of those great sieves, the kidneys.
- is the perfect liquid for the blood.
- is the ideal liquid for efficient functioning of the lungs, stomach, liver and all other vital organs.
- is universally accepted as the standard for biomedical applications and for drinking water purity.
- is so pure that all drug prescriptions are formulated with distilled water.
- is fresh, clean and pleasing to the palate.
- makes foods and drinks prepared with it taste noticeably better. The flavor is subtle enough not to interfere with the food it is mixed with.
- is the only pure water left on our polluted planet!
- is the healthiest water and is the greatest natural solvent on earth!

Prevention is Always Better than a Cure

Although most seldom realize it, they live continually under the fear of sickness and death. They would even indignantly deny this assertion and insist that they are not afraid to die – although most of us are willing to admit the fear of developing some deadly physical condition that may make us a less efficient human than we are now.

People always fear the unknown: for that very reason we have learned to expect catastrophes from many unanticipated sources. But if we fully understand what disease is and how it originates and if we become familiar with the only avenues through which illness can strike us, then what have we to fear except ourselves?

To prevent disease is to circumvent the daily cause of illness . . . which, as previously discussed, is the clogging of our bodies with deadly chemicals and inorganic minerals, salt and the increasing amounts of toxic, acid by-products of digestion and metabolism – all conditions which we can control by our lifestyle.

So, if we can recover from disease by a reversal of our wrong habits of living, won't these same good habits prevent disease in the first place? Prevention may cost little, but it sure saves a lot! If one is of sound mind, it must seem clear that the only sane method is to avoid an unhealthy lifestyle that causes disease. Prevention is the best way to feel and remain youthful, energetic and virile throughout a long, healthy life.

If we are to prevent disease, we must have a rudimentary knowledge of our bodies. Our bodies are composed of millions of cells bathed in an electrolytic solution consisting of organic calcium, magnesium, potassium, sodium and phosphorus, etc., with trace amounts of copper and zinc. These are all organic minerals. The body cannot use inorganic minerals for building its cells. These electrolytes are held in solution by water, which makes up 70% of the body. For this reason, we can live without food for long periods, but we can only live about 72 hours without water. So you can see how important it is that the body not only gets sufficient water, but the right kind of water. Distilled water is absolutely necessary for super health!

The vast majority of people drink ordinary tap water laced with chemicals and inorganic minerals. The body can make no selections for itself, but must accept what you put into it. When you give the body water that is heavily loaded with chemicals and inorganic minerals, the body has to do something with these poisons. It therefore stores them in your arteries, veins, joints, eyes, ears, nose, throat, gallbladder and other vital organs.

Our Bodies Can Only Endure So Much Severe Punishment and Still Survive!

Because the body is such a wonderful instrument, it can take a great deal of punishment and still function. For many years the body seems to handle the situation. But the day finally arrives when the poisons you have loaded into your body begin to give you trouble – real trouble: increasing pain, suffering, misery and agony!

127

Those people who have laughed in Mother Nature's face now cry out in pain, "Help me! Save me from my terrible suffering!" These are the people who want a cure. A cure? No one can cure you of anything!

Only the basic biological functions of the body can perform a cure. Don't wait until pain strikes to start taking care of your wonderful body! It may be too late then. Today is the day to outline a health program for yourself and live by it faithfully hereafter.

You get only one body during your lifetime. If you want to live in health and freedom from suffering, you must faithfully follow the Health Laws of Mother Nature. These are good, kind laws. She wants you to have a painless, tireless, ageless body. It is your birthright to feel the thrill of joyous living every day of your life!

I have treated with only water well over 3,000 persons with dyspeptic pain. They all responded to an increase in their water intake, and their clinical problems associated with the pain disappeared. – F. Batmanghelidj, M.D.

By following Mother Nature's great and good laws you can awaken one beautiful morning to discover the feeling of radiant health and happiness! You'll have slept deeply like a baby. Gone are your headaches, gone is your chronic fatigue, gone are all your aches and pains! You'll feel new vitality surging throughout your entire body. You'll have a spring in your step, a sparkle in your eyes and the glow of health in your skin. You'll have found the greatest and most precious treasure in the whole world – radiant, glorious health! Physical and mental health are now yours!

Perpetual Youthfulness Can Be Yours!

Longfellow says that "In youth the heart exults and sings!" This suggests the idea that beyond certain prescribed years the heart does not exult and sing.

Youth, in its crudest sense, does not refer to years but to a state of being. It really is a matter of one's own choice, if one is born with a normal constitution, as to when youth shall end and "middle age" begin. Some people can truly be referred to as youthful although they may have seen fifty or more years.

Every normal person really desires to remain youthful, but few are willing to pay the price. The price of prolonged youthfulness is the consistent faithful performance of certain healthy lifestyle habits.

These healthy lifestyle habits are: staying away from chemicalized drinking water full of inorganic minerals; eating no salt; drinking ample amounts of distilled water only; eating a well-balanced and natural diet; consistent and proper exercise; deep power breathing; good personal hygiene; and thinking positively. Without a healthy body, one cannot maintain positive thinking!

You now know that the most destructive force that robs you of youthful good health consists of a gradual settling of insoluble inorganic mineral matter from water and salt into the tissues of your body. This encrustation begins first on the walls of the arteries, gradually diminishing their elasticity and caliber as well as the nourishment of the tissues they supply. As a consequence

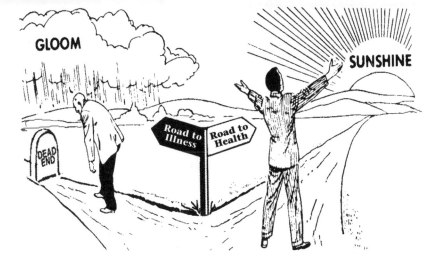

GLOOM

SUNSHINE

Road to Illness

Road to Health

DEAD END

The choice of which road to take is up to the individual. He alone can decide whether he wants to reach a dead end or live a healthy, wholesome, long, happy, active life. – Paul C. Bragg

129

of these destructive changes, all body functions slow down more and more until some vital organ stops altogether and death occurs from premature ageing. The beginning of corrosion and the subsequent hardening of the arteries are the first stages of premature ageing, no matter how long a person has lived!

Your life-long work is the battle to keep your arteries free from the inorganic minerals and chemicals contained in most drinking water. Stop using table salt and eat a balanced diet that does not leave a residue of toxic crystals to clog and obstruct your circulation.

You now know what we know . . . the shocking truth about water . . . and what we believe to be the world's best-kept health secret. Let's really make life a healthful, vigorous adventure! Health and happiness are our goals. Health is our wealth! There are no failures possible for those who start today and move steadily onward in their quest for perfect, youthful health!

To maintain good health, the body must be exercised properly (stretching, walking, jogging, running, biking, swimming, deep breathing, good posture, etc.) and nourished wisely (with natural foods), so to maintain a normal weight and increase the good life of radiant health, joy and happiness. – Paul C. Bragg

Bragg Blessings to you our Health Friend!

Our sincere blessings to you, our dear friends, who make our lives so worthwhile and fulfilled by reading our teachings on the healthy lifestyle of living that our Creator laid down for us all to follow. Yes, He wants us all to follow the simple path of natural living and this is what we teach through our worldwide Health Crusades and books. Our prayers reach out to you, wishing the best in health and happiness to you and your loved ones. This is the birthright He promised us all, but we must follow the laws He has laid down for us, so that we can reap this precious health physically, mentally and spiritually!

Paul C. Bragg   *Patricia Bragg*

Man's days shall be to 120 years. – Genesis 6:3

UNCOMPLICATE YOUR LIFE

Life is a continual lesson in problem solving,
but the trick is to know where to start. No excuses!
Start your Bragg Healthy Lifestyle today!

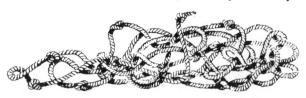

I never suspected that I would have to learn how to live – that there were specific disciplines in ways of seeing the world that I had to master before I could awaken to a simple, healthy, happy, uncomplicated life. – Dan Millman

What a person eats and drinks becomes his own body chemistry.

Vitamin E is now known as the primary defender against free radical damage. Since stores of this nutrient decline with age, it is important to supplement your diet with vitamin E-rich foods such as wheat germ, nuts, green leafy vegetables and polyunsaturated vegetable oils.

Chapter 7

SPECIAL SUPPLEMENT

Since its first publication, *Water – The Shocking Truth* has been in such demand that the 27th printing of the book was almost sold out the day it was printed! This book, we feel, played an important part in the development of the widespread public awareness of Mother Earth's environmental problems. Man is finally realizing that he cannot continue to contaminate this planet Earth and survive. This newly revised Special Supplement will bring you the latest and most important information on this vital subject.

A New Era of Personal Ecology

The damage to our natural resources has become personalized in the form of a terrible threat to our health and our very lives. Technology has outstripped biology! The increasing mechanization and industrialization of our society – at first welcomed as benefactors bringing creature comforts and labor-saving devices – are now revealed as "Trojan Horses" bringing the various enemies into our very homes to destroy us!

131

Biochemists Shocked by Lab Tests

Biochemists are alarmed by the result of laboratory tests which reveal increasing deposits of inorganic "heavy metals" in our bodies. The dangerous effects of the increasing pollution of our water, soil, food and air are evidenced by the fact that:

- 90% of tests show mercury poisoning.
- 85% of tests show lead intoxication.
- 37% of tests show arsenic poisoning.
- 70% of tests show zinc accumulations.

SHOCKING FACTS: Fluoride is more toxic than lead. Levels of fluoride in water are 67 times higher than permissible lead levels. – Health Action Network

Poisoned By Food and Water

Mercury . . . lead . . . arsenic . . . zinc . . . none of us deliberately take these inorganic mineral poisons into our systems. Or do we? How could we? Health-minded people drink distilled water, fruit and vegetable juices, and eat organic foods.

The tragic truth about the water and organic foods and juices is that even these substances can become contaminated, because so much of our air, water and soil are contaminated by industrial and agricultural pollutants. We are aware of radioactive fallout and have demanded safeguards against it. But what about the daily fallout of inorganic wastes from factory chimneys? What about poisonous pesticides, chemical fertilizers and deadly food additives?

Rain water, for example, was once and rightly considered pure – but no longer! Pure it may be when it leaves the clouds. But after it passes through air polluted by industrial and automotive wastes – including everything from sooty carbons to strontium, arsenic, selenium, beryllium, copper, lead, mercury and fluorides – it should be labeled "hazardous to your health!"

When these poisons, especially the deadly fluoride gases, are absorbed by the soil it also becomes toxic. Add to this the contaminants contained in poisonous pesticides and chemical fertilizers that large industrial farms and growers use to increase crop production. Grains, vegetables and fruits will absorb these poisons and so will meat from animals that feed on contaminated grass and fodder. Is it any small wonder that so many people are only half-alive?

Amino Acids are Vital to Life

From the smallest germ cell of life to the most complicated living organism, amino acids are now recognized as the activating ingredients of life itself. Amino acids are responsible for the production of proteins; the building blocks of the body; as well as the hormones and enzymes responsible for thinking and memory, breathing and muscle action.

The Biological Sciences have isolated some 30 distinct varieties of amino acids. Most of these are manufactured within our bodies, but some must be supplied daily by the food we eat. These amino acids are essential to life – life cannot exist without them!

Heavy Metals Murder Amino Acids

The discovery of amino acids was a tremendous scientific breakthrough. Now we are on the threshold of another – the unmasking of the murderer of these amino acids which are so essential to life. The substances which lead to the destruction of the body chemicals necessary for the metabolizing and manufacturing of these vital amino acids are proving to be – you guessed it! – inorganic heavy metals from industrial and agricultural contaminants.

"Plastic" Food Removes Vital Amino Acids

Trace organic minerals are also vital to the production of amino acids by the body. By natural law, these are supplied directly by fruit, vegetables and grains. Today, however, we are being robbed of these essential elements. No trace organic minerals can be found in the "plastic," demineralized, devitalized foods produced from depleted soils that are deadened and contaminated further by the use of inorganic fertilizers and pesticides. The end result is lifeless supermarket produce with good "eye appeal" but little or no nutritional value.

Protective Action in Personal Ecology

With inorganic heavy metal toxicity caused by air and water pollutants, and a loss of the essential daily supply of trace minerals due to contaminated and depleted soil, it is not surprising that many tests are revealing a dangerously low count of amino acids.

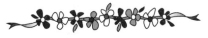

I have found a perfect health, a new state of existence, a feeling of purity and happiness, something unknown to humans!
– Novelist Upton Sinclair, a frequent faster

What Can We Do to Protect Ourselves?

These actions can be taken now, while we wait for more information on these important discoveries:

1. Learn more about amino acids and the enzymes that make them work, and the poisons that can kill them.

2. Have your health practitioner administer:
    a) tests for mercury, arsenic, lead, fluorides, strontium and all heavy metals.
    b) the comparatively new test known as "30 amino acids fractionation test."

3. Encourage your friends and loved ones to seek the assistance of their doctors in measuring their bodies for these substances before they become problematic, therefore causing diseases.

4. Make sure that the source of your organic food is in an area free from airborne pollution and grown in soil enriched by only natural fertilizers.

5. Follow the precepts of this book in regard to your drinking water! Drink only steam-distilled water.

Political Action for Permanent Ecology

During recent years, in response to heightened public opinion, politicians have promised in their political platforms action in solving our ecological problems. Millions of dollars have been spent on studies, and volumes of words printed and spoken.

But the ever-increasing problems of pollution and a dangerously disrupted ecology are still plaguing us. The air in our cities is fast approaching or exceeding crisis conditions. Our drinking water sources – our rivers, lakes and ocean shorelines – are becoming contaminated far beyond established safe levels.

Scientific bodies and institutions throughout the world agree that we are in danger of self-extinction unless we stop abusing our vital life-support systems. They have offered sober warnings and countdown time tables. So far these warnings have received but token hearings from governmental and political ears.

But there is one voice that every politician heeds – the combined voice of aroused voters who demand action! This is the one sound that rises above the clink of campaign contributions from big industrial, agricultural, manufacturing, financial and business interests. To achieve the desired effect – political action on any and all levels – the voice of the voters must be strong, widespread and united in purpose.

What Can One Person Do?

Whether you are counting to 10 or to a million, you have to begin with one! That's how political action starts. Begin with yourself, your family, your friends and neighbors, involve your clubs, your church and other groups, write letters to the editor of your local newspaper. Call and write your local radio and TV stations. Go to town council meetings and state your concerns.

After you get your hometown or community involved, extend your action into the county . . . the state . . . the nation! Write, visit and call county officials, state officials and your congressmen and women, and even the President and Vice-President of the United States! Don't settle for promises or palliatives! Demand action – and persist until you get it!

135

It is up to each and every one of us to bring all possible political pressure to bear upon our political leaders to clean up our environment and restore the world's natural ecology. This is what we must do – it is our responsibility – if we hope to see the 21st Century!!

Let's Clear Up Some Confusion

On the basic issues of pollution and ecology, practically all health-minded persons agree. On other issues among ourselves, however, there seems to be some disagreement. On the subject of nutrition, for example, there was so much controversy among the advocates of various diets – each claiming theirs was the only one worthwhile – that we felt it necessary to clarify matters. As the world's oldest practicing biochemist and nutritionist, with personal experience in evaluating the numerous and varied dietetic theories, my father has shared his great knowledge with all those who are interested in our revealing, life-changing book, *Bragg Healthy Lifestyle – Vital Living to 120*. (See back pages to order this book if unavailable in your area.) Now water, and its safety, has become a similar controversy.

What is "Pure Water"?

Reading this book, *Water – The Shocking Truth That Can Save Your Life,* you are becoming aware of the pros and cons of distilled water versus mineral or ground water. Unfortunately, however, writers and lecturers are now creating confusion about distilled water. Some have actually referred to "soft water" (water treated by a water softener) as "distilled water." This is definitely not the case! Softened water has a high content of inorganic sodium, calcium and other inorganic minerals.

Using this misinformation as a basis, even some health publications have made misleading comparisons in an attempt to make a case against distilled water! For example, group comparisons were made citing people who lived in remote areas with hard ground water supplies and yet had a low incidence of cardiovascular (heart and circulatory system) problems – without also taking into consideration the pertinent fact that such people tend to eat more natural "live" foods and live in a relaxed, rural environment!

On the basis of water alone, this rural group was compared with people living in crowed, highly polluted metropolitan areas who drank treated city water, presumably filtered through home water softeners (erroneously designated as "distilled water"), who showed a higher incidence of hypertension and other cardiovascular problems. No mention was made of the obvious facts that these urban dwellers were subjected to much greater tensions, as well as diets of lifeless, processed "plastic" foods from supermarket shelves – both major contributors to cardiovascular illnesses.

Obviously, any self-styled "researcher" who makes such errors as those noted above has not done their basic homework! Unfortunately, the reader may not be aware of this – and thus unnecessary confusion is irresponsibly created. So, with water as with eating, don't let the "experts" fool you!

What is Distilled Water?

Throughout this book we have stressed that distilled water is the only pure water – the only water you should put into your body. As noted previously, "soft water" is not distilled water . . . nor is "purified water," "deionized water," "filtered water" or "reverse osmosis water."

There is only one process that can make 100% distilled water and that is steam distillation. In steam distillation, only pure water (H_2O) evaporates, leaving all inorganic minerals and other impurities behind.

Drinking Safe Water

With so many of our public water supplies contaminated by harmful chemicals and toxic additives, how can we make sure that we provide only safe, healthful water for ourselves and our families? One relatively simple answer is to drink only distilled bottled water. But even this method requires care, for not all bottled water lives up to even FDA bottled water standards. Before you buy any bottled water ask for an analysis – it's your right and it's your health at risk! Let's work to prevent these water atrocities and get quick action to clean up our country's precious water supplies!!! Call or write to your bottled water company and your city water board to demand proof that your water supply contains no THMs (trihalomethanes, also formed through chlorination), carcinogens, fluoride and other synthetic or organic chemicals and pesticides! Get your water tested! Call your local Public Health Department for details and cost.

Associated Press, 2/11/98 – The EPA is set to unveil new requirements that will provide citizens with details on what chemicals are found in their drinking water. President Clinton said the new water quality reports are necessary "to ensure that Americans have the information they need about the safety of their drinking water." The new EPA regulation will direct water agencies nationally to provide information such as: • What lakes, underground aquifers or rivers the water comes from. • What contaminants are in the water and whether the amounts exceed EPA health standards. • What health risks are posed by the contamination when federal standards are exceeded.

How Drinking Water Affects Your Health

Pure water is a necessity for health! In research begun way back in 1960, the water supplies of 1,633 of the largest cities in the U.S. were analyzed. Results of this long study showed a definite link between water quality and the mortality rate from cancer, cardiovascular disease and other chronic diseases.

TDS and Chronic Disease

In his study, "Relationship of Water to the Risk of Dying," Dr. Sauer chronicled the relationship of Total Dissolved Solids to heart disease, cancer and other chronic diseases (Total Dissolved Solids – or TDS – is the term for all the elements present in any water supply). It had been thought for centuries that the European mineral waters so very high in TDS were beneficial to health. But Dr. Sauer's study found that as TDS increases in a water supply, so does the number of chronic diseases in the population using that supply.

(Author's Note: At our home in Desert Hot Springs, one of California's renowned hot mineral water resorts, our water pipes had to be replaced after only a few years due to mineral buildup in the pipes. What this inorganic mineral-laced water does to the plumbing in buildings it also does to human pipes!)

High Blood Pressure and Drinking Water

Water quality also plays a part in the development of hypertension, or high blood pressure. Hypertension afflicts over 50 million people in the U.S., making it the most common chronic disease. It is also a major health problem in all of the developed countries of the world – due to stress, the introduction of refined foods, salt, lack of exercise, and water dehydration.

But the good news about hypertension, or high blood pressure, is that it can be reduced or even prevented! A diet high in natural fiber, grains, vegetables, organic calcium and potassium – with less meat, fat and sodium – can help reduce or even prevent hypertension.

It's estimated that fully 10% of our sodium intake is from drinking water! A study of high school sophomores in a community with high levels of sodium in their drinking water showed significantly higher blood pressure levels than those in areas with less sodium in their water. The girls among this first group had blood pressure patterns characteristic of persons 10 years older! Follow up studies in the same area among even younger children, ages 7 to 11 years, produced similar results.

The conclusion from this and other studies seems obvious: increased sodium levels in drinking water leads to increased blood pressure levels. The American Heart Association, the EPA (Environmental Protection Agency) and the World Health Organization – among other health groups – recommend that sodium levels in drinking water should not exceed 20 mg/liter. And yet, of 2,100 water supplies included in a survey by the U.S. Public Health Service, 42% had sodium ion concentrations above this level! About 5% showed levels greater than 250 mg/liter!

Water Softeners + Sodium = Trouble

We have already seen the strong relationship between soft water and heart disease! But that is only part of the story – for softened water also poses grave health risks in terms of hypertension.

The usual method for softening water is to add 2 parts sodium which then extracts 1 part calcium and 1 part magnesium from the water supply. This results in "softer" water which is higher in sodium. So it would seem that the "luxury" of having soft water to bathe in and for laundry is hardly worth the increased risks to health and longevity!

The Sad Truth About Chlorination

Water chlorination has been widely used to "purify" water in this country for most of this century. But its negative effects on health surely outweigh any benefits.

Dr. Joseph Price, for one, believes that there is a definite link between widespread chlorination of water supplies and the increasing incidence of heart disease! In the animal experiments he conducted, chlorine caused atherosclerosis in 95% of the animals tested!

Chlorine in the water supply has been linked with cancers of the bladder, liver, pancreas and urinary tract in certain areas. To take just one example of what is happening around the world, in New Orleans the drinking water is taken from the Mississippi River. Over 66 new carcinogenic compounds have been isolated in that city's water supply as a result of adding chlorine – a substance which naturally combines with methanol, carbon disulfide and other compounds! A very high incidence of colon cancer has been found in this city.

Cancers and Chlorination

An investigator at the government's National Cancer Institute, Kenneth Cantor, points out that many studies since the early 1974 report on New Orleans have confirmed its findings, linking increased carcinogens in the water supply to additional cancer deaths annually. Cantor and his associates completed a study of nearly 3,000 men and women who had been drinking chlorinated water in such cities as New York, Chicago, Atlanta, Detroit, New Orleans, San Francisco and Seattle. Subjects were also studied in Connecticut, Iowa, New Jersey, New Mexico and Utah. This study conclusively linked bladder cancer to drinking chlorinated water.

Nor is the risk limited to bladder cancer alone. Theresa Young of the Department of Preventive Medicine at the University of Wisconsin led a study to determine the effect of chlorinated water on women. She checked the death certificates of women in Wisconsin who had died from cancers of the gastrointestinal system, the urinary tract, brain, lungs and breast.

The kind of water you drink can make or break you – your body is 70% water!

Ample evidence points to chlorine-based chemicals as significant contributors to breast cancer.
– Thornton, *Breast Cancer and The Environment: The Chlorine Connection*

The major finding was that colon cancer in women was "significantly associated" with exposure to water which was disinfected with low, medium and high daily chlorine doses for at least 20 years. She said her study should be examined in the context of the theory linking colon cancer to a high fat, low fiber diet. She also stated that researchers should pursue other theories of colon cancer as well – such as industrial pollutants and chlorine-induced carcinogens in drinking water.

One expert, Dr. Herbert Schwartz, is quite emphatic in asserting that "chlorine is so dangerous it should be banned." He believes that chlorine-treated water alone is directly responsible for cancer, heart disease and premature senility!

Can Miscarriages and Birth Defects Be Caused by Tap Water?

A recent 5,000 woman, one million dollar study conducted by the State of California revealed that women who drank tap water had twice as many miscarriages and children born with birth defects as those who drank bottled water or had filtering devices on their taps. Five large studies have come to the same conclusion, according to State Health Director Kenneth Kizer. Only two aspects of health were addressed by these studies. It is impossible even to guess how many other ailments affecting men, women and children and pets can be directly attributed to tap water.

Dangerous Chemicals In Our Drinking Water

There is more and more evidence that the majority of human cancers are environmental in origin and thereby largely preventable. In fact, an astounding number of chemical – and possibly carcinogenic – compounds are found in our water supplies after treatment and in surface and ground water sources.

A recent ABC News exposé revealed the shocking fact that over 700 chemicals have already been found in our drinking water! Of these, 129 have been pinpointed by the EPA as posing serious health risks. Yet that same agency requires that our water supplies be regularly tested for only 14 of them!

One carcinogen found in many municipal water systems, chloroform, can be introduced during chlorine treatment. A known animal carcinogen, it is present in measurable levels in nearly all municipal water systems as a by-product of water chlorination!

Fluoride and Cancer

Fluoride is among the most potentially dangerous of all water additives. Long-term research into fluoridation has shown that its positive effects on dental health are minimal at best and are far outweighed by the serious health risks resulting from its use. Cancer researcher Dr. Dean Burke believes that 10% of all cancer deaths in the U.S. may be due directly to fluoridation! Yet, 40% of the citizenry continues drinking fluoridated water. Dr. Burke and his associate, Dr. John Yiamouyiannis, have concluded that drinking fluoridated water may increase your risk of dying from cancer by 5% to 15%!

Home Water Distillation & Filtration Systems

The best method of ensuring a safe water supply is to install a home water distillation system. A filtration system, changing filters often, can purify your tap water, but, as with bottled water, filtration systems must be evaluated and consumer lab reports given careful study. Some systems remove up to 99% of THMs and synthetic organic compounds. All less efficient systems provide a false sense of security to consumers. (Filtered water is NOT distilled water.) We've researched the processes and equipment available for making distilled water. We will continue to review and experiment with new equipment as it comes on the market. Please see water system comparison chart on page 165. For information on the best home water distillers available see resource page 166.

Dehydration of certain organs will result in symptoms which are often mis-diagnosed by physicians. The message is: drink your way to health with volumes of pure water. – F. Batmanghelidj, M.D. author of
  Your Body's Many Cries for Water; You Are Not Sick, You Are Thirsty!

Deadly Chemical Cocktails

Dr. Joseph Price, famous U.S. medical researcher and author of the book *Coronaries/Cholesterol/Chlorine* stated "Chlorine is the greatest crippler and killer of modern times. Two decades after the start of chlorination of our drinking water system in 1904, the present epidemic of heart disease and cancer began."

Fluoride has a voracious appetite for the enzymes that help you with correct digestion, thereby reducing your body's ability to absorb the vitamins essential for good health. While the debate continues, some authorities believe that fluoride may cause birth defects, genetic damage, cancer and allergic responses. More immediately apparent is dental fluorosis, a gross mottling of young people's teeth. If fluoride can mottle teeth, what does it do to your skeletal system, etc.? Former Department of Health Principal Dental Officer, Dr. John Colquhoun, was one of the instigators of fluoridation in New Zealand. However, after much research, seeing the toxic long-term effects of fluoride consumption, he is now one of the foremost opponents of fluoridation.

The Human Cell is Immortal

Dr. Alexis Carrel, brilliant scientist at the Rockefeller Institute, won the greatest award, the Nobel Prize in medicine by demonstrating his arresting hypotheses: *the Cell is Immortal*. It is merely the fluid in which it floats that degenerates. Renew the fluid at regular intervals, give the cells what they require for nutrition and as far as we know, the pulsation of life may go on forever. His hypotheses was that, premature death and many symptoms of the ageing process are due to an accumulation of toxins in the cells of the body. These toxins are from cellular decay and also enter your body in the air you breathe, the food you eat and the water you drink. This overload of toxins keeps your body from absorbing and utilizing the nutrition that your cells so desperately need. According to Dr. Carrel, if your cells are cleansed of all toxins and the proper nutrients are provided, you should be able to live without ageing.

Since your body is about 70% water, the blood and lymphatic system over 90% water, it's essential for your health you consistently drink only pure water that's not saturated with contaminants, inorganic minerals and toxins. This water will transport vital nutrients to cells and waste from cells more efficiently. This allows the body to function correctly and stay healthier!

Organic Minerals Are Essential to Health

ORGANIC MINERALS. Your minerals must come from an organic source, from something living or that has lived. Humans do not have the same chemistry as plants. Only the living plant has the ability to extract inorganic minerals from the earth and convert them to organic minerals for your body to absorb and utilize.

INORGANIC MINERALS. Inorganic minerals and toxic chemicals in water can create these problems:

144

- Clog and harden the veins, capillaries and arteries.
- Harden the liver.
- Cause kidney and gallstones.
- Cause arthritis, bone spurs and painful calcified formations in the joints.
- Inorganic minerals and toxic chemicals in water clog the arteries and small capillaries that are needed to feed and nourish your brain with oxygenated blood; the result is loss of memory and gradual senility and strokes.

AVERAGE TAP WATER INGREDIENTS:
Chlorine, fluoride, arsenic, lead, cadmium, aluminum, copper, trihalomethanes, calcium carbonate, chloroform, unpleasant taste.

Cocktail of Toxic Chemicals

The California Safe Drinking Water Initiative, to be on the ballot in California June 1998, reads: The public water supply should be safe for all to drink. In order to protect the public health from increased risk of hip fracture, cancer, dental fluorosis and other harmful effects which have been linked to fluoride in the scientific literature, and whereas data from the U.S. Public Health Service and the State of California show no significant difference in decay rates of permanent teeth and dental costs in fluoridated and nonfluoridated areas in California; Section 116410 of the Health and Safety Code is amended to read: No fluoride or fluoride-containing substance may be added to public water systems. All laws to the contrary are hereby repealed. Urge Californians and everyone to read this book – it's a health alert for sure!

> **Distilled water is nature's health tonic and is free of inorganic minerals and toxic chemicals. You will enjoy drinking it, drink it more often and bloom!**

- Water regulates all body functions. It is essential for the removal of wastes, especially from body tissues.

- Water stops skin from wrinkling, leaving it clear, healthy and resilient. You will actually look younger.

- Water helps to maintain a healthier muscle tone.

- Distilled water will help you lose weight. It suppresses the appetite naturally.

- Drinking lots of distilled water is the best treatment for fluid retention, for it helps remove toxins.

- Distilled water helps banish constipation, aiding the body to rid itself of wastes efficiently and regularly.

Drinking 8 to 10 glasses of distilled water daily is the master key to health and vigor. It's a preventative to help protect us from this poisonsous industrial age. It's a vital fluid that helps keep our bodies in better health.

145

Distilled Water Acts as a Natural Cleansing Solvent in the Body

The purer water is (free from inorganic minerals, dissolved heavy metals, softeners, pollutants, etc.) the more toxins it can absorb and carry out of the body; also, the more nutrients it will be able to carry to the body's cells. Other fluids made from water like coffee, alcohol, tea, cola drinks, etc. are already heavily saturated with toxins and are less able to absorb and carry away toxins. Incredible as it may seem, water is quite possibly the single most important catalyst in losing weight and keeping it off. Although most of us take it for granted, water may be the only true 'magic potion' for permanent weight loss. It's usually best not to drink beverages with meals, as it dilutes the digestive enzymes. Drink water up to ½ hour before or not less than ½ hour after meals.

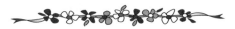

Let food be your medicine, and medicine be your food. – Hippocrates

Pure Water is the Greatest Life-Giver!

Pure water is truly one of God's greatest gifts to us, a source of life and health. Making sure that we use only water that is safe and uncontaminated (distilled is best) may be one of the greatest health gifts we can give ourselves, our families and friends! Distilled water is the world's best and purest water! It is excellent for detoxification and fasting programs and for cleaning of all the cells, organs and fluids of the body because it helps carry away so many harmful substances!

Water from chemically-treated public water systems – and even from many wells and springs – is likely to be loaded with poisonous chemicals and toxic trace elements! Depending upon the kind of piping that the water has been run through, the water in our homes, offices, schools, hospitals, etc., is likely to be overloaded with zinc (from old-fashioned galvanized pipes) or with copper and cadmium (from copper pipes). These trace elements are released in large quantities by the chemical action of the water on the metals of the pipes.

146

Pure Water – Essential for Health

Whether it be from the natural juices of vegetables, fruits and other foods or from the water of high purity obtained by steam distillation, pure water is essential for health. Your body is constantly working for you . . . breaking down old bone and tissue cells and replacing them with new ones. As the body casts off the old minerals and other waste products of broken-down cells, it must obtain fresh supplies of the essential elements for new cells. Scientists are only now beginning to understand how various kinds of dental problems, different types of arthritis and even some forms of hardening of the arteries are caused by the various kinds of imbalances in the levels of calcium, phosphorus and magnesium in the body's chemistry. Disorders can also be caused by imbalances in the ratios of minerals.

Each individual healthy body requires a proper balance within itself of all the nutritive elements. It is just as bad for an individual to have too much of one item as it is to have too little of another one. It takes appropriate levels of phosphorus and magnesium to keep calcium in solution so that it can be transformed into new cells of bone and teeth. Yet, there must not be too much of those nutrients, nor too little calcium in the diet, or old bone will be taken away but new bone will not be formed. In addition, we now know that diets which are unbalanced and inappropriate for a given individual can deplete the body of calcium, magnesium, potassium and other major and minor elements.

Diets which are high in meats, fish, eggs, grains, nuts, seeds and their products may provide unbalanced excesses of phosphorus which will deplete calcium and magnesium from the bones and tissues of the body, causing those minerals to be lost in the urine. A diet high in fats will tend to increase the intake of phosphorus from the intestines relative to calcium and other basic minerals. Such a high-fat diet can result in the loss of calcium, magnesium and other basic nutrients in much the same way a high-phosphorus diet does.

147

Diets excessively high in fruits or their juices may provide unbalanced excesses of potassium in the body, and calcium and magnesium will again be lost from the body through the urine. These deficiencies of calcium and magnesium can produce all kinds of problems in the body, ranging from dental decay and osteoporosis to muscular cramping and twitching, hyperactivity, poor sleep patterns, and excessive frequency and uncontrolled patterns of urination. Similarly, deficiencies of other minerals or imbalances in the levels of those minerals can produce many other problems.

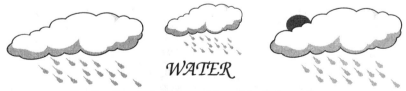

WATER

To the days of the aged it addeth length;
To the might of the strong it addeth strength;
It freshens the heart, it brightens the sight;
'Tis like quaffing a goblet of morning light.

Despite numerous dietary sources such as these, many adults and children in so-called civilized cultures will be found to have low levels of essential minerals in their bodies due to losses caused by drinking coffee, tea, and carbonated beverages, combined with the long-term habit of eating bad, "plastic" foods containing too much sugar and table salt, as well as products made from refined flours. In addition, the body's organs can be thrown out of balance by continued stress, toxins in our air and water, along with disease-produced injuries or pre-natal deficiencies linked to the mother's unhealthy diet or lifestyle. As a result many, if not most, people in our so-called civilization may need to take a natural chelated multiple mineral supplement as well as a broad-range multiple vitamin for extra insurance.

Therefore, it is important to clean and detoxify the body through fasting and drinking only pure distilled water as well as organically-grown vegetable and fruit juices. At the same time, it is also important to provide the body with an adequate source of new minerals. This can be done by eating a variety of healthy organic vegetables, including kelp and other sea vegetables for adults and natural healthy mother's milk for infants.

Warning – Milk and it's Dangers!

We do not recommend using animal milks, specifically cow's milk, for several reasons. First, almost all milk is pasteurized (boiled). Milk that is not labeled raw has been boiled to kill all bacteria so you don't get sick from drinking it. Bacteria is not the only thing that is killed during boiling. Pasteurized milk is dead. If anything is left alive, the homogenization process destroys it. Why would you want to drink dead milk?

Milk also contains an enzyme called lactose which most people are allergic to. The major symptom of a lactose allergy is mucus formation. Many people think lots of mucus and handkerchiefs, nose-blowing and tissues are just a normal part of life. But they're not! These people haven't realized that they are lactose intolerant. If they stopped consuming milk and other dairy products, most would find themselves drastically reducing their mucus production and use of tissues.

You must take into consideration all of the herbicides, pesticides and fungicides that cattle ingest through their feed. These toxins are passed on to you through their milk. This is to say nothing of all the hormones, growth stimulators, antibiotics and other drugs that are pumped into cattle to treat disease and maximize weight and milk production. These chemicals and poisons also make their way into the milk. As far as raw milk is concerned, remember that the reason that pasteurization became mandated by law was because so many people were dying from bacterial diseases that they contracted from drinking raw milk.

And what about the cattle industry's policy of feeding cows the rendered (ground-up) remains of other cows? How healthy do you think the milk of a cannibal cow really is? Also, if you think these cattle are given distilled water to drink, you need to visit a feed lot and see for yourself. You would be appalled at the conditions!

In short, if you value your health, you should abstain from consuming milk and all of its products: cheese, buttermilk, sour cream, cream cheese, eggnog, cream, half and half, butter, yogurt, ice cream and even whey, which most people don't realize is a milk protein.

> ***When not hungry, don't eat!***
> ***Make your body earn and desire its nourishment***
> ***with vigorous activity, exercise and work!***

The word "vegetarian" is not derived from "vegetable," but from the Latin, homo vegetus, meaning among the Romans "a strong, robust, thoroughly healthy man." – Paul C. Bragg

Happiness is not being pained in body or troubled in mind. – Thomas Jefferson

Steam distillation is an extremely effective method of guarding against waterborne mirco-organisms because such contaminants cannot vaporize.

Skin Absorbs Water, Toxins and All!

*Compared with its absorption through the respiratory system, skin absorption could be the major route of penetration into the body. Skin penetration rates have been found to be remarkably high, and the outer layer of skin is a less effective barrier to penetration than traditionally assumed. Factors affecting absorption are:

Hydration: The more hydrated the skin, the greater the absorption. If the skin is hydrated (through perspiration or immersion in water) or if the contaminant compounds are in solution, diffusion and penetration will be enhanced.

Temperature: Increased skin or water temperature will enhance skin absorption capacity proportionately. During swimming and bathing, it may be expected that greater hydration of skin surfaces will take place.

Skin Condition: Any insult (i.e. sunburn) or injury (i.e. cuts, wounds, abrasions) to the skin will lower its ability to act as a barrier against foreign substances. A history of skin disease such as psoriasis or eczema acts to lower the natural barrier of the outer skin layer, as do rashes, dermatitis, or any chronic skin condition.

Regional Variability: Skin absorption rates vary with the different regions of the body. Underestimated is the case of whole body immersion during swimming or bathing. The epidermis of the hand represents a relatively greater barrier to penetration than many other parts of the body, including the scalp, forehead, abdomen, area in and around the ears, underarms and genital area. Penetration through the genital area is estimated to be 100% but only 8.6% for the forearm.

Other Routes of Entry: Other significant routes of absorption include oral, nasal, cheeks and mouth cavity, and eye and ear areas. These routes have been underestimated in their ability to absorb contaminants during immersion in water. Inhalation serves as yet another route. In the case of swimming or bathing, the

---

More men fail through lack of purpose than lack of talent. – Billy Sunday

volatilized chemicals are likely to gather near the surface of the water and are readily inhalable. In addition, some of the water may be swallowed in these situations.

–*From *the American Journal of Public Health*

You Get More Toxic Exposure from Taking a Shower Than From Drinking the Same Water!

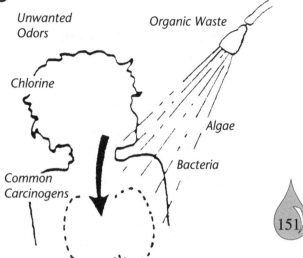

*Two of the very highly volatile and toxic chemicals, trichloroethylene and chloroform have been proven as contaminants in most municipal drinking-water supplies. The great National Academy of Sciences has estimated that 200 to 1,000 people die in the United States each year from the cancers caused largely by ingesting water pollutants from inhalation as air pollutants in the home. Inhalation exposure to water pollutants has largely been ignored. Data indicates that hot showers can liberate about 50% of the chloroform and 80% of the trichloroethylene into the air.

Tests show that your body can absorb more chlorine as a result of a 10-minute shower than if you drank 8 glasses of the same water. How can that be?

A warm shower opens up your pores, causing your skin to act like a sponge. As a result, you not only inhale the chlorine vapors, you absorb them through your skin, directly into your bloodstream – at a rate that's up to 6 times higher than drinking it.

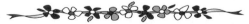

To help retard the processes of premature and decrepit old age, it is essential that you drink plenty of distilled water daily.
– Dr. N.W. Walker, *Water Can Undermine Your Health*

In terms of cumulative damage to your health, showering in chlorinated water is one of the most dangerous risks you take daily. Short-term risks include: eyes, sinuses, throat, skin and lung irritation. Long-term risks include: excessive free radial formation (that ages you faster!), higher vulnerability to genetic mutation and cancer development, difficulty metabolizing cholesterol which can cause hardened arteries.

– * From Science News

Five Hidden Dangers in Your Shower:

• **Chlorine:** Added to all municipal water supplies, this disinfectant hardens arteries, destroys proteins in the body, irritates skin and sinus conditions and aggravates any asthma, allergies and respiratory problems.

• **Chloroform:** This powerful by-product of chlorination causes excessive free radical formation (accelerated ageing!), normal cells to mutate and cholesterol to form. It's a known carcinogen!

• **DCA (Dichloroacedic acid):** This chlorine by-product alters cholesterol metabolism and has been shown to cause liver cancer in lab animals.

• **MX (another chlorinated acid):** Another by-product of chlorination, MX is known to cause genetic mutations that can lead to cancer growth and has been found in all chlorinated water for which it was tested.

• **Proven cause of bladder and rectal cancer:** Research proved that chlorinated water is the direct cause of 9% of all US bladder cancers and 15% of all rectal cancers.

Showers, Toxic Chemicals & Chlorine

Skin absorption of toxic contaminants has been underestimated and ingestion may not constitute the sole or even primary route of exposure.

– Dr. Halina Brown, *American Journal of Public Health*

Taking long hot showers is a health risk, according to the latest research. Showers – and to a lesser extent baths – lead to a greater exposure to toxic chemicals contained in water supplies than does drinking the water. These toxic chemicals evaporate out of the water and are inhaled. They can also spread through the house and be inhaled by others. People receive 6 to 100 times more chemicals by breathing the air around showers and baths than they would by drinking the water.

– Ian Anderson, *New Scientist*

A professor of Water Chemistry at the University of Pittsburgh claims that exposure to vaporized chemicals in the water supplies through showering, bathing, and inhalation is 100 times greater than through drinking the water.   – *The Nader Report – Troubled Waters on Tap*

Chlorine is the greatest crippler and killer of modern times. While it prevented epidemics of one disease, it was creating another. Twenty years after the start of chlorinating our drinking water in 1904, the present epidemic of heart trouble, cancer and senility began.

– Dr. Joseph Price, *Coronaries/Cholesterol/Chlorine*

Don't Gamble With Your Health – Use a Shower Filter

The most effective method of removing these hazards from your shower is the quick and easy installation of a filter on your shower arm. The filter we found to be the best removes chlorine, lead, mercury, iron, chlorine by-products, arsenic, hydrogen sulfide, and many other unseen contaminants, such as bacteria, fungi, dirt and sediments. It has a 12 to 18 month filter life-span and the filter can be easily cleaned by backwashing and replaced when needed. It comes with a money-back guarantee. To get the best shower filter call 800-446-1990. I have been using this filter for 3 years and really enjoy my chlorine-free showers! Now you can order one, too!

Start enjoying safe, chlorine-free showers right away. It's essential to reducing your risk of heart disease and cancer and to ease the strain from your immune system. And you may even get rid of long-standing conditions – from sinus and respiratory problems to dry, itchy skin.

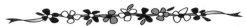

You can save yourself much money and the anxiety of falling ill by paying attention to your body's constant need for pure water.
– Dr. F. Batmanghelidj, *Your Body's Many Cries For Water*

Total Health for the Total Person

In a broad sense, "Total Health for the Total Person" is a combination of physical, mental, emotional, social and spiritual components. The ability of the individual to function effectively in their environment depends on how smoothly these components function as a whole. Of all the qualities that comprise an integrated personality, a well-developed, totally fit and healthy body is the most desirable.

A person may be said to be totally physically fit if they function as a total personality with efficiency and without pain or discomfort of any kind. It means having a Painless, Tireless, Ageless Body that possesses sufficient muscular strength and endurance to maintain an effective posture; successfully carry out the duties imposed by one's environment; meet emergencies satisfactorily; and enough energy for recreation and social obligations after the "work day" has ended. The Total Person's body also meets the requirements for his environment through efficient functioning of sensory organs, possesses the resilience to recover rapidly from fatigue, stress and strain without the aid of stimulants; enjoys natural sleep at night and wakes feeling fit and alert in the morning, prepared for the day ahead.

154

Keeping the body totally fit, healthy and in excellent working order is no job for the uninformed or careless person. It requires an understanding of the body, sound health and eating practices and living a disciplined healthy lifestyle. The results of such a regimen can be measured in happiness, radiant health, agelessness, peace of mind and high achievement in the joy of living.

Paul C. Bragg   Patricia Bragg

Good Health, generated by physical fitness, is the logical starting point for the pursuit of excellence in any field. Physical vitality promotes mental vitality and thus is essential to executive achievement.
– Dr. Richard E. Dutton

Ten Common-Sense Reasons Why You Should Only Drink Pure, Distilled Water!

- There are over 12,000 chemicals on the market today . . . and 500 are being added annually! Regardless of where you live – in the city or on the farm, some of these chemicals are getting into your drinking water.

- No one knows what effects these toxic chemicals may have upon the body and what and how many toxic combinations are created. It's like making a mixture of colors; one drop can change the color.

- No equipment has been designed to detect these harmful chemical combinations and may not be for years.

- The body is made up of approximately 70% water, the essential fluid of life. Therefore, don't you think you should be wise about the type of water you drink?

- The Navy has been drinking distilled wter for years!

- Distilled water is chemical and mineral free. Distillation removes all the chemicals and impurities from water that are possible to remove. If distillation doesn't remove them, there is no method known today that will.

155

- The body does need minerals, but it's not necessary that they come from water. There is not one mineral in water which cannot be found more abundantly in food! Water is the most unreliable source of minerals because it varies from one area to another. The food we eat – not the water we drink – is our best reliable source of organic minerals!

- Distilled water is used for intravenous feeding, inhalation therapy, prescriptions and baby formulas. Therefore, doesn't it make common sense that distilled water is good and healthier for everyone?

- Thousands of water distillers have been sold throughout the United States and many foreign countries to individuals, families, dentists, doctors, hospitals, nursing homes and government agencies . . . and these informed, alert consumers are helping protect their health by using only pure distilled water.

- With all of the chemicals, pollutants and other impurities in our water, it only makes good common sense that you should clean up the water you drink the inexpensive way, through distillation.

Chlorination of water supplies is sufficient reason in itself to drink and shower in pure distilled water. – Harvey & Marilyn Diamond, *Fit for Life*

Praises for: *Water – The Shocking Truth*

"In my opinion, *Water – The Shocking Truth* is destined to become a landmark – not just in the field of so-called health literature – but particularly in the field of standard internal medicine. Following a massive coronary thrombosis 13 years ago, I have been on a strict regimen of distilled water, health diet, vitamin therapy and exercise – and the results have exceeded my expectations. I feel better at 67 than I did at 47. My arteries are clean and healthy; my joints have limbered; my vision is sharper; my nerves are calmer; and my head is clearer. My own experience corroborates your findings. I am convinced that distilled water has been the most important facet of my rejuvenation program."

– Ben H. Martin, Lakewood, CA

"Thank you for your fine review of my books, *Hunza Land* and *The Choice Is Clear*. And let me repeat my thanks to you for your great book, *Water – The Shocking Truth*, which I recommend as a 'must' to all my patients. In connection with this subject, I would like to emphasize that a vital factor in the amazing longevity of the people of Hunza Land is distilled water. They eat most of their fruits and vegetables raw, raised in organic soil. Fruits and vegetables, of course, are 90% distilled water – nature's own distillation, as you say. Along with that, they drink glacier water, which is low in inorganic minerals. Their main beverage is an organic grape drink, which again is distilled water. So, in isolated Hunza Land, the intake of distilled water is 90% greater than that of our overrated western civilization."

– Allen E. Banik, O.D., Kearney, NE

"I have read your book, *Water – The Shocking Truth*, and find it indeed shocking. Thank you for the enlightenment. This should be required knowledge in every medical school and health-related field."

– Chris R. Linville, M.D., New Brunswick, NJ

"Your book on water is a masterpiece!"
–H. Rosenthal, Richmond Hill, Ontario, Canada

Praises for: *Water – The Shocking Truth*

"For the past few years I have been doing research work on hardening of the arteries and related poblems of ageing. Your book, *Water – The Shocking Truth*, is the best and most reasonable I've read on this subject."
– Betty Watts, Pasadena, CA

"I belong to a Health Club in Buffalo, N.Y., and our members all agree that your shocking wonderful book on water is the best book on the market. Thank you!"
– H.W. Hoffman, Hamburg, NY

"One of the greatest things that ever happened to me was attending your health classes 35 years ago in Miami, Florida. Thanks to your teachings, I am now 57 years young and love living The Bragg Healthy Lifestyle!! I have read all of the Bragg books many times, and have just finished the sixth reading of your *Water* book. To me this is the greatest book! Keep up the crusading!"
– Cliff Hayes, Deerfield Beach, FL

157

"I have been on distilled water for about five months, ever since I read your book. I had pains in my knuckles and a calcium deposit on my left shoulder. These have all left me now; also my bowel elimination is a lot better."
– C.A. McFeaters, Hainesville, PA

"As outlined in your book, *Water – The Shocking Truth*, I know that the closer to nature we can get, the better off we are going to be . . . I am a farmer in Missouri, and have not used any chemicals of any kind on this farm for 15 years, as I came to realize that we should not try to improve on nature, but work with her! I am so happy to find people like you and Patricia, who are not trying to keep the truth to yourselves. You are true health crusaders leading people toward healthy long lives."
– Eugene Kling, Meadville, MO

"From start to finish, this is the most inspiring book on water and health I've had the pleasure of reading!"
– Mrs. Elizabeth Risch, Ridgefield, NJ

Questions and Answers

Q. *Water – The Shocking Truth,* **is so informative that I wish to give copies of it to my children, their families and all of our friends. Do you offer a special price on a dozen or more copies?**

A. Yes, there is a special rate on the purchase of a dozen or more copies of any Bragg publication. In fact, many church groups, service clubs and school organizations buy Bragg Books in quantity lots for individual resale at regular prices for their fund-raising projects.

Q. **Will distilled water help my complexion?**

A. Yes – distilled water will help you have a smooth, firm, radiant complexion in 2 ways – by drinking it for internal cleanliness and by cleansing your skin with it externally. Hard water seals the pores and tends to clog them. For thorough, healthful cleansing, use distilled water on your skin. Distilled water is an excellent hair rinse and leaves hair soft.

Q. **I have an obesity problem. Will drinking distilled water help me to lose weght?**

A. First, eliminate salt from your diet. A primary symptom of obesity is retention of fluid. A major cause of waterlogged tissues is due to the fact that table salt, composed of sodium chloride, is an inorganic mineral which is indigestible by the human body and is held in solution with water. Hard water makes this condition worse by adding more indigestible inorganic minerals, further impairing the body's system of elimination. Pure, distilled water will help your body to function at its best in

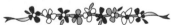

Fasting is an effective and safe method of detoxifying the body, a technique that wise men have used for centuries to heal the sick. Fast regularly and help the body heal itself and stay well.
– Dr. James Balch, Prescription for Nutritional Healing

It's magnificent to live long if one keeps healthy and youthful. – Harry Fosdick

Nothing transforms anyone as much as changing from a negative to a positive attitude.

every way, including the better elimination of accumulated harmful inorganic substances. Distilled water is especially good for your liver and kidneys, which are the organs most abused by salt and hard water, inorganic minerals, fluorides, chlorides, etc.

Q. What is your opinion of the honey and vinegar treatment for arthritis advocated by Dr. Jarvis?

A. It's an excellent treatment – except he should have specified distilled water. * A ¼ cup raw, organic apple cider vinegar added to gallon of distilled water, flavored with raw honey – a drink fit for the gods – and helps you feel like one! Remember, it took years to build-up your arthritic condition, so don't expect overnight clean-up miracles. Work with Mother Nature and be as patient as she is with you. * For more vinegar miracles read the Bragg Vinegar Book.

Q. Is distilled water recommended for babies?

A. Yes, it's not only recommended, it's prescribed for babies! Distilled water should be used internally, also externally for cleaning babies. Diaper rash and skin problems can result from hard water deposits and chemicals even on sheets, clothes, cotton & wool diapers, etc. Do final rinse in distilled water.

Q. Can animals and wildlife tell the difference between hard and distilled water?

A. Yes. Place a variety of waters before a goat, for example, and he will select distilled water. Use it in your bird bath and the birds will return yearly. Many a race has been lost because trainers didn't provide their thoroughbreds with distilled water.

Q. Does hard water affect everyone the same way?

A. No. All human systems are basically similar, but no two are exactly alike! Mineral deposits from hard water tend to migrate to the body's weakest points: the intestinal walls, causing constipation; the kidneys, creating stones; in the arteries, leading to arteriosclerosis; in the joints, inviting arthritis; etc.

There is no wealth greater than the health of the body. – Bible

Of course, when the functions of any one part of the body are impaired, the entire system is affected and gradually weakened. Thus, multiple symptoms appear as evidence of more widespread systematic damage. Your best insurance against all these symptoms of "ageing" is to drink distilled water.

Q. Do athletes drink distilled water?

A. The wise ones do. Connie Mack, 30 years Yankee mgr, would not allow his players to drink hard water on any occasion – and he had champion healthy teams. Connie Mack also "practiced what he preached" and maintained his own perfect health past 90. We have lots of champion teams in all sports and olympic and triathlete champions as well as the Dallas Cowboys who follow the Bragg Healthy Lifestyle and drink pure distilled water!

Q. We have recently installed a home water softener. Dr. Bragg, is this good, pure drinking water?

A. Don't drink it! Water softeners do not eliminate inorganic minerals, but merely hold them in suspension in an ionized state. It makes more soapsuds – but leaves inorganic mineral deposits in your home and human plumbing to cause problems!

Urgent Health Alert!

Thousands of gallons of the potentially deadly gas additive methyl tertiary butyl ether – or MTBE – are leaking every day into our precious water supplies from underground storage tanks across the United States! This chemical, which is purported to reduce car emissions and is mandated by Federal law is suspected of causing a wide range of diseases including asthma, nosebleeds and cancer. It has even appeared in the pristine water of Lake Tahoe! **Act now!** *Call or write your government representatives today! Join your local chapter of an action group (like OxyBusters, Greenpeace or the Sierra Club) before this 3 billion dollar a year cash cow pollutes our water forever.*

As the tide of chemicals born in the Industrial Age has arisen to engulf our environment, a drastic change has come about in the nature of the most serious public health problem. For the first time in the history of the world, every human being is now subject to contact with dangerous chemicals, from the moment of conception until death. – Rachel Carson, Silent Spring, 1962
It's sad the world did not follow our friend's wise warnings in her landmark book. We could have saved billions of wildlife that needlessly died plus humans that have lost their lives to deadly chemicals pesticides, herbicides, etc. – P.B.

Recommended – Water Research Reading

Alhava, E. M., et al, *The effect of drinking water fluoridation on the fluoride content, strength and mineral density of human bone*, Acta Orthop Scand 51:413-20, 1980.

Arnala, I., *Bone fluoride, histomorphometry, and incidence of hip fracture*, University of Kuopio, 1983.

Avioli, L.V., *Fluoride treatment of osteoporosis, Postgraduate Medicine: A special report*, pp. 26-7, September 14, 1987.

Burgstahler, A. W. and Colquhoun, J., *Neurotoxicity of fluoride*, Fluoride 29:57-8, 1996.

Chlebna-Sokol, D. and Czerwinski, E., *Bone structure assessment on radiographs of distal radial metaphysis in children with dental fluorosis*, Fluoride 26:3744, 1993.

Cohn, P. D., *A brief report on the association of drinking water fluoridation and the incidence of osteosarcoma among young males*, New Jersey Department of Health, November 8, 1992.

Colquhoun, J., *Disfiguring dental fluorosis in Auckland, New Zealand*, Fluoride 17:66-72, 1984.

Cooper, C., Wickham, C. A. C., Barker, D. J. R. and Jacobsen, S. J., *Water fluoridation and hip fracture*, Journal of the American Medical Association 266:513, 1991.

Czerwinski, E., et al, *Bone and joint pathology in fluoride-exposed workers*, Archives of Environmental Health 43:340-3, September/October 1988.

Danielson, C., Lyon, J. L., Egger, M. and Goodenough, G. K., *Hip fractures and fluoridation in Utah's elderly population*, Journal of the American Medical Association 286:746-8, 1992.

Diesendorf, M., *The mystery of declining tooth decay*, Nature 322:125-9, 1986.

Erickson, *Mortality in selected cities with fluoridated and nonfluoridated water supplies*. New England Journal of Medicine, 298:1112-6, 1978.

Fejerskov, O., Manji, F. and Baelu, V., *The nature and mechanisms of dental fluorosis in man*, Journal of Dental Research 69:692-700, 1990.

Foulkes, R. G., *Case report: mass fluoride poisoning, Hooper Bay Alaska, etc.*, Fluoride 27:32-36, 1994.

Foulkes, R. G. and Anderson, A., *Impact of artificial fluoridation on salmon species in the U.S. Northwest and British Columbia*, Canada, Fluoride 27:220-6, 1994.

Freni, S. C., *Exposure to high fluoride concentration in drinking water is associated with decreased birth rates*, Journal of Toxicology and Environmental Health 42:109-121, 1994.

Gessner, B.D., Beller, M., et al, *Acute fluoride poisoning from a public water system*, New England Journal of Medicine 330; 2:95-99, 1994.

Gibson, S. L. M., *Effects of fluoride on immune system function*, Comp Medical Research 6:1111-13, 1992.

Hedlund, L. R. and Gallagher, J. C., *Increased incidence of hip fracture in osteoporotic women treated with sodium fluoride*, Journal of Bone and Mineral Research 4:223-5, 1989.

Jacobsen, S. J., et al, *Regional variation in the incidence of hip fracture*, Journal of the American Medical Association 264:500-502, 1990.

Hip fracture incidence before and after the fluoridation of the public water supply, Rochester, Minnesota, American Journal of Public Health 83:743-5, 1993.

Kalsbeek, H., Verrips, G. H. W., *Dental caries prevalence and the use of fluorides in different European countries*, Journal of Dental Research 69:728-32, 1990.

Leverett, D. H., *Prevalence of dental fluorosis in fluoridated and nonfluoridated communities – preliminary investigation*, Journal of Public Health Dentistry 46:184-7, 1986.

Madams, et al, *The relationship between hip fracture and water fluoridation: an analysis of national data*, American Journal of Public Health 81:475-9, April 1991.

Mahoney, M. C., et al, *Bone cancer incidence rates in New York State: time trends and fluoridated water*, American Journal of Public Health 81:475-9, April 1991.

Masuda, T. T., *Persistence of fluoride from organic origins in waste waters*, Devel. Indust. Microbiology 5:53-70, 1964.

Munzenberg, K. J., Moller, F. and Kock, W., *Adverse effects of osteoporosis treatment with fluoride*, Munchener Medizinische Wochenshrift, 133(5):56-8, 1991.

Schnitzler, C. M., et al, *Bone fragility of the peripheral skeleton during fluoride therapy for osteoporosis*, Clinical Orthopaedics and Related Research 261:268-71, 1990.

Scott, F., Editorial, *Fluoridation: more evidence it is not safe or effective*, American Laboratory, June 1986.

Smith, G., *A surfeit of fluoride?* Science Pro, Oxford, 69:429-42, 1985.

Sowers, F. R., et al, *The relationship of bone mass and fracture history to fluoride and calcium intake: a study of three communities*, American Journal of Clinical Nutrition 44:889-98, 1986.

A prospective study of bone mineral content and fracture in communities with differential fluoride exposure, American Journal of Epidemiology 133:649-60, 1991.

Susheela, A. K., et al, Fluoride ingestion and its correlation with gastrointestinal discomfort, Fluoride 25: 5-22, 1992.

Sutton, P. R. N., *Fluoridation, Errors and Omissions in Experimental Trials*, Melbourne University Press, 1959 & 1960.

U.S. Department of Health and Human Services, Agency for Toxic Substances and Disease Registry, *Toxicological Profile for Fluorides, Hydrogen Fluoride, and Fluorine* (F), April 1993.

Waldbott, G. L. and Lee, J. R., *Toxicity from repeated low-grade exposure to hydrogen fluoride - case report*, Clinical Toxicology 13:391-402, 1978.

Weingrad, T. R., et al, *Periostitis due to low-dose fluoride intoxication demonstrated by bone scanning*, Clinical Nuclear Medicine 16:59-61, 1991.

163

Yiamouyiannis, J., *Water fluoridation and tooth decay: results from the 1986-1987 National Survey of U.S. school children*, Fluoride 23:55-67, 1990.

Fluoridation and cancer: the biology and epidemiology of bone and oral cancer related to fluoridation, Fluoride 26:83-96, 1993.

Zhao, L. B., et al, *Effect of a high fluoride water supply on children's intelligence*, Fluoride 29:190-2, 1996.

Fluoride, The Aging Factor, 3rd Ed., by John Yiamouyiannis, Ph.D. Health Action Press, 6439 Taggart Road, Delaware, Ohio 43015, 1993.

The Fluoride Question - Panacea or Poison? by Anne-Lise Gotzsche. Stein and Day, Scarborough House, Briarcliff Manor, New York , NY 10510, 1975.

"Fluoridation of Water," a special report by Bette Hileman, Chemical and Engineering News; 66(31):26-42, 1988.

Fluoride: The Freedom Fight by Hans Moolenburgh, M.D. Mainstream Press, Edinburgh, 1987.

Fluoride in Australia: A Case to Answer by Wendy Varney. Hale and Iremonger, GPO Box 2552, Sydney, NSW, Australia, 1986.

Fluoridation in New Zealand by Bruce Collins. New Zealand Pure Water Association, Box 2186, Tauranga, New Zealand.

The Greatest Fraud, Fluoridation by Phillip R. N. Sutton, D.D.S. Kurunda Pty. Ltd., Box 22, Lorne, Australia 3232, 1996.

"Fluoridation: Commie Plot or Capitalist Ploy?" by Joel Griffiths, Covert Action, Fall 1992.

"Celebration or Shame? Fifty Years of Fluoridation (1945-1995)" by Richard G. Foulkes, Townsend Letter for Doctors and Patients, November 1995.

"Analyzing the Fluoridation Controversy" by Brian Martin in Social Studies of Science, Vol. 18 (1988) pp. 331-63 (SAGE Publications, 2111 West Hillcrest, Newberry Park, CA 91320).

Scientific Knowledge in Controversy: The Social Dynamics of the Fluoridation Debate by Brian Martin, State University of New York Press, Albany, New York, 1991.

Comparison of Water Treatment Technologies

POLLUTANT	Filter Sediment	Filter Carbon	Deionization	Reverse Osmosis	Steam Distillation
Arsenic	○	○	●	●	●
Bacteria	○	○	○	◐	●
Cadmium	○	○	●	●	●
Calcium	○	○	●	●	●
Chlorides	○	○	●	●	●
Chlorine	○	●	○	●[1]	●[1]
Cryptosporidium	○	○	○	●	●
Detergents	○	◐	●	●	●
Fluorides	○	○	●	●	●
Lead	○	○	●	●	●
Magnesium	○	○	●	●	●
Nitrate	○	○	◐	◐	●
Organics	○	●	○	●[1]	●[1]
Pesticides	○	●	○	●[1]	●[1]
Phosphates	○	○	●	●	●
Radon	○	○	●	●	●
Sediment	●	◐	●	●	●
Soduim	○	○	●	●	●
Sulfates	○	◐	●	●	●
Viruses	○	○	○	○	●

○ Ineffective or No Reduction　◐ Significant Reduction　● Complete or Significant Reduction

1 – A Carbon Filter Needed (The best home distillers have carbon filters.)

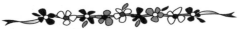

For more info on water distillers for your home & shower head filters
to remove harmful chemicals from your shower water
please see the resource page on 166.

165

PROMISE YOURSELF

- *To be so strong that nothing can disturb your peace of mind.*
- *To talk health, happiness, prosperity to every person you meet.*
- *To make all your friends feel that they are special.*
- *To look at the sunny side of everything and make your optimism come true.*
- *To think only of the best, work only for the best and expect only the best.*
- *To be just as enthusiastic about the success of others as you are about yours.*
- *To forget the mistakes of the past and press on to the greater achievements of the bright, fresh future.*
- *To wear a cheerful countenance at all times and give every living creature you meet a smile.*
- *To give so much time to the improvements of yourself that you have no time to be critical of others.*
- *To be too large for worry, too strong for fear, too noble for anger, and too happy to permit the presence of trouble.*

– Christian D. Larson

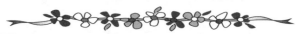

Your posture carries you through life from your head to your feet. This is your human vehicle and you are truly a miracle! Cherish, respect and protect it by living The Bragg Healthy Lifestyle. – Patricia Bragg

The nervousness and peevishness of our times are chiefly attributable to tea and coffee. The digestive organs of confirmed coffee drinkers are in a state of chronic derangement which reacts on the brain, producing fretful and lachrymose moods. – Dr. Bock, 1910

Drinking 8 glasses daily of pure distilled water cleanses and recharges the human batteries! – Paul C. Bragg

The chlorine in your shower water is a powerful toxin – and slowly can poison your body! – Kathleen Peddicord, What Doctors Don't Tell You

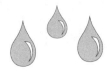 # Index

167

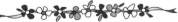

Prayer is the mortat that holds our house together. – Sister Teresa

Men do not die; they kill themselves. – Seneca, Roman Philosopher

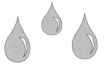
Index
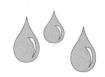

168

Distillation effectively removes the widest variety of contaminants from water. – David & Anne Frahm, *Healthy Habits*

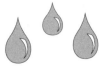

Index

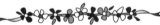

There is only one water that is 100% clean and that is steam distilled water. No other substance on our planet does so much to keep us healthy and get us well as this water does. – Dr. James F. Balch, MD, *Dietary Wellness*

The greatest domestic problem facing our country is saving and keeping our soil and water healthy for our unborn generations ahead.
– Senator Sam Rayburn, Washington, D.C.

The best system to purify water is distillation, which boils the water into steam to kill organisms . . . and also remove impurities.
– Boardroom Reports Inc., *The Great Book of Health Secrets*

Distillation effectively removes the widest variety of contaminants from water. – David & Anne Frahm, *Healthy Habits*

Jesus said, "Thy faith hath made thee whole, now go and sin no more." That includes your dietetic sins! He himself, through fasting and prayer, was able to heal the sick and cure all manner of diseases.

FROM THE AUTHORS

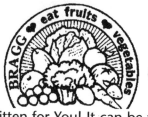

GO ORGANIC

This book was written for You! It can be your passport to the Good Life. We Professional Nutritionists join hands in one common objective – a high standard of health for all and many added years to your life. Scientific Nutrition points the way – Mother Nature's Way – the only lasting way to build a body free of degenerative diseases and premature ageing. This book teaches you how to work with Mother Nature, not against her. Doctors, nurses, and professional care givers who care for the sick try to repair depleted tissues, which too often mend poorly – if at all. Many of them praise the spreading of this message of natural foods and methods for long-lasting health and youthfulness at any age. This book was written to speed the spreading of this tremendous message.

Statements in this book are recitals of scientific findings, known facts of physiology, biological therapeutics and reference to ancient writings as they are found. Paul C. Bragg practiced the natural methods of living for over 80 years with highly beneficial results, knowing that they were safe and of great value. His daughter Patricia Bragg worked with him to carry on the Health Crusades. They make no specific claims regarding the effectiveness of these methods for any individual, and assume no obligation for any opinions expressed in this book.

No cure for disease is offered in this book. No foods or diets are offered for the treatment or cure of any specific ailment. Nor is it intended as, or to be used as, literature aimed at promoting any food product. Paul C. Bragg and daughter Patricia express their opinions solely as Public Health Educators and Health Crusaders.

Experts may disagree with some of the statements made in this book, particularly those pertaining to nutritional recommendations. However, such statements are considered to be factual, based upon the long-time experience of Paul C. Bragg and Patricia Bragg. If you suspect you have a medical problem, please seek alternative health professionals to help you make the healthiest, wisest and best-informed choices.

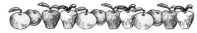

Bragg Blessings to You, Our Treasured Friends

From the Bragg home to your home we share our years of health knowledge – years of living close to God and Mother Nature and what joys of fruitful, radiant living this produces – this my Father and I share with you and your loved ones. With Love and Blessings for Health, Peace and Happiness. – Patricia

Bragg Organic Raw Apple Cider Vinegar
With the Mother . . . Nature's Delicious, Healthy Miracle

HAVE AN APPLE HEALTHY DAY!

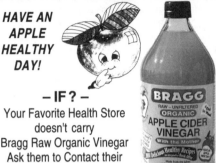

– IF ? –

Your Favorite Health Store doesn't carry Bragg Raw Organic Vinegar Ask them to Contact their Health Distributor to stock it! Or they can Call Bragg at 1-800-446-1990

BRAGG RAW – UNFILTERED **ORGANIC** **APPLE CIDER VINEGAR** With the Mother **IN GLASS BOTTLES**

INTERNAL BENEFITS:
- Rich Miracle Enzymes & Potassium
- Natural Antibiotic & Germ Fighter
- Helps Control & Normalize Weight
- Improves Digestion & Assimilation
- Helps Fight Arthritis & Stiffness
- Relieves Sore & Dry Throats
- Helps Remove Toxins & Sludge

EXTERNAL BENEFITS:
- Helps Promote Youthful, Healthy Body
- Helps Promote & Maintain Healthy Skin
- Soothes Sunburn, Shingles & Bites
- Helps Prevent Dandruff & Itchy Scalp
- Soothes, Aching Joints & Muscles

BRAGG APPLE CIDER VINEGAR

SIZE	PRICE	USA SHIPPING & HANDLING	AMT	$ TOTAL
16 oz.	$ 2.19 ea.	Please add $3 for 1st bottle and $1.50 each additional bottle		.
16 oz.	$ 24.09	Case/12 S/H Cost by Time Zone: CA $7. PST/MST $8. CST $12. EST $14.		.
32 oz.	$ 3.79 ea.	Please add $4 for 1st bottle and $2.00 each additional bottle.		.
32 oz.	$ 41.69	Case/12 S/H Cost by Time Zone: CA $10. PST/MST $14. CST $20. EST $24.		.

Bragg Vinegar is a food and not taxable

Foreign orders, please inquire on postage.

Please Specify: ☐ Check ☐ Money Order ☐ Cash

Charge To: ☐ Visa ☐ MasterCard ☐ Discover

Credit Card Number:

Total Vinegar $	.
Shipping & Handling	.
Total Enclosed $ (USA Funds Only)	.

Month Year

Card Expires:

MasterCard **VISA** **DISCOVER** **Signature:**

CREDIT CARD ORDERS ONLY
CALL **(800) 446-1990**
OR FAX **(805) 968-1001**

Business office calls (805) 968-1020. We accept MasterCard Discover or VISA phone orders. Please prepare your order using this order form. It will speed your call and serve as your order record. Hours: 9 am to 4 pm Pacific Time, Monday thru Thursday.
Visit our Web Site: http://www.bragg.com & e-mail: bragg@bragg.com

Mail to: **HEALTH SCIENCE, Box 7, Santa Barbara, CA 93102 USA**

Please Print or Type – Be sure to give street & house number to facilitate delivery.

V-BOF-803

Name

Address   Apt. No.

City   State

Phone (   )   • Zip

Bragg Apple Cider Vinegar – Taste You Love, Health You Need!
Available Health Stores - Nationwide

BRAGG ALL NATURAL LIQUID AMINOS

Delicious, Healthy Seasoning Alternative to Tamari & Soy Sauce

BRAGG LIQUID AMINOS — Nutrition you need...taste you will love...a family favorite for over 85 years. A delicious source of nutritious life-renewing protein from soybeans only. Add to or spray over casseroles, soups, sauces, gravies, potatoes, popcorn, and vegetables. An ideal "pick-me-up" broth at work, home or the gym. Gourmet health replacement for Tamari and Soy Sauce. Start today and add more Amino Acids to your daily diet for healthy living — the easy BRAGG LIQUID AMINOS Way!

SPRAY or DASH brings NEW TASTE DELIGHTS! PROVEN & ENJOYED BY MILLIONS.

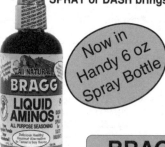

Now in Handy 6 oz Spray Bottle

Spray or Dash of Bragg Aminos Brings New Taste Delights to Season:
- Salads
- Dressings
- Soups
- Veggies
- Tofu
- Rice/Beans
- Tempeh
- Stir-frys
- Wok foods
- Gravies
- Sauces
- Meats
- Poultry
- Fish
- Popcorn
- Casseroles & Potatoes
- Macrobiotics

Pure Soybeans and Pure Water Only
- No Added Sodium
- No Coloring Agents
- No Preservatives
- Not Fermented
- No Chemicals
- No Additives

BRAGG LIQUID AMINOS

SIZE	PRICE	USA SHIPPING & HANDLING	AMT	$ TOTAL
6 oz.	$ 2.98 ea.	Please add $3 for 1st 3 bottles – $1.25 each additional bottle.		
6 oz.	$ 68.54 Case/24	S/H Cost by Time Zone: CA $5. PST/MST $7. CST $9. EST $11.		
16 oz.	$ 3.95 ea.	Please add $3 for 1st bottle – $1.25 each additional bottle.		
16 oz.	$ 43.45 Case/12	S/H Cost by Time Zone: CA $6. PST/MST $7. CST $10. EST $11.		
32 oz.	$ 6.45 ea.	Please add $4 for 1st bottle – $1.50 each additional bottle.		
32 oz.	$ 70.95 Case/12	S/H Cost by Time Zone: CA $8. PST/MST $11. CST $16. EST $19.		

Bragg Liquid Aminos is a food and not taxable

Foreign orders, please inquire on postage

Please Specify: ☐ Check ☐ Money Order ☐ Cash

Charge To: ☐ Visa ☐ MasterCard ☐ Discover

Total Aminos	**$**
Shipping & Handling	
Total Enclosed (USA Funds Only)	**$**

Credit Card Number: _ _ _ _ — _ _ _ _ — _ _ _ _ — _ _ _ _   Card Expires: ___ Month ___ Year

Signature: _____

CREDIT CARD ORDERS ONLY
CALL **(800) 446-1990**
OR FAX **(805) 968-1001**

Business office calls (805) 968-1020. We accept MasterCard Discover or VISA phone orders. Please prepare your order using this order form. It will speed your call and serve as your order record. Hours: 9 am to 4 pm Pacific Time, Monday thru Thursday.
Visit our Web Site: http://www.bragg.com & e-mail: bragg@bragg.com

Mail to: **HEALTH SCIENCE, Box 7, Santa Barbara, CA 93102 USA**

Please Print or Type – Be sure to give street & house number to facilitate delivery.

A-BOF- 803

Name _____

Address _____ Apt. No. _____

City _____ State _____

Phone (___) _____ Zip _____

Bragg Aminos – Taste You Love, Nutrition You Need!
Available Health Stores - Nationwide

BRAGG "HOW-TO, SELF-HEALTH" BOOKS

Authored by America's First Family of Health
Live Longer – Healthier – Stronger Self-Improvement Library

Qty.	Bragg Book Titles ORDER FORM Health Science ISBN 0-87790	Price	$ Total
_____	**Apple Cider Vinegar — Miracle Health System**	6.95	•
_____	**The Bragg Healthy Lifestyle - Vital Living to 120** (Formerly Toxicless Diet)	7.95	•
_____	**Super Power Breathing for Super Energy – High Health & Longevity**	7.95	•
_____	**Miracle of Fasting** (Bragg Bible of Health for physical rejuvenation & longevity)	8.95	•
_____	**Water – The Shocking Truth** (learn safest water to drink & why)	7.95	•
_____	**Nature's Healing System to Improve Eyesight** in 90 days (foods, exercises, etc.)	7.95	•
_____	**Bragg's Complete Gourmet Recipes** for Vital Health – 448 pages	8.95	•
_____	**Bragg Health & Fitness Manual** – Triathlon Manual – Swim-Bike-Run – for All Ages		•
	A Must for Athletes, Triathlete & would-be-athletes – 600 pages	16.95	•
_____	**Build Powerful Nerve Force** (reduce stress, fear, anger, worry)	7.95	•
_____	**Keep Your Heart & Cardiovascular System Healthy & Fit** at Any Age	7.95	•
_____	**Nature's Way to Reduce** (lose 10 pounds in 10 days)	6.95	•
_____	**Hair and Your Health**, Nature's Way to Beautiful Hair (easy-to-do method)	7.95	•
_____	**Sauerkraut & Cabbage Recipes** Raw, Salt-Free (make your own – it's so healthy)	2.95	•
_____	**Healthy, Strong Feet** – "Best Complete Foot Progam" – Dr. Scholl	7.95	•
_____	**Fitness/Spine Motion** – For a More Flexible, Pain-free Back	3.95	•
_____	**Nature's Way to Health** (simple method for long, healthy life to 120)	6.95	•

Total Copies Prices subject to change without notice.

TOTAL BOOKS $ •

USA Shipping Please add $2.00 for first book, $1.00 for each additional book.
USA retail book orders over $35.00 add $5.00 only.
Canada & Foreign orders add $2.00 per book.

CA residents add sales tax •

Shipping & Handling •

Please Specify: ☐ Money Order ☐ Cash ☐ Check

Charge To: ☐ Visa ☐ Master Card ☐ Discover

TOTAL ENCLOSED $ •
(USA Funds Only)

Month Year

Credit Card Number: ___ ___ ___ ___ — ___ ___ ___ ___ — ___ ___ ___ ___ — ___ ___ ___ ___   Card Expires: _____ |

Signature: _____

Please Print or Type – Be sure to give street & house number to facilitate delivery.
BOF- 803

• _____
Name

• _____
Address   Apt. No.

• _____
City   State

Phone (_____) _____   • Zip _____

Send for Free Health Bulletins

Let Patricia Bragg send you, your relatives and friends the latest discoveries on Health, Nutrition, Exercise and Longevity. These are sent free periodically. All donations and gifts are tax deductible and appreciated for our spreading the gospel of health to everyone, including schools, churches, prisons and institutions, etc. Also, your donations will help fund our planned Health Retreats which are needed now more than ever! For more information please see page ii up front.

With Blessings of Health and Thanks,

Patricia

Please print or type addresses clearly . . .

BRAGG HEALTH CRUSADES, Box 7, Santa Barbara, CA 93102

●
_____
Name

_____ (____) _____
Address   Phone

_____
City   State   Zip Code

●
_____
Name

_____ (____) _____
Address   Phone

_____
City   State   Zip Code

●
_____
Name

_____ (____) _____
Address   Phone

_____
City   State   Zip Code

●
_____
Name

_____ (____) _____
Address   Phone

_____
City   State   Zip Code

●
_____
Name

_____ (____) _____
Address   Phone

_____
City   State   Zip Code